Innovative Prosthetic Device

Innovative Prosthetic Device

New Materials, Technologies and Patients' Quality of Life (QoL) Improvement

Editors

Marco Cicciù
Luca Fiorillo
Rosa De Stefano

MDPI • Basel • Beijing • Wuhan • Barcelona • Belgrade • Manchester • Tokyo • Cluj • Tianjin

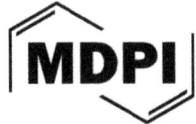

Editors
Marco Cicciù
Department of Biomedical and
Dental Sciences, Morphological
and Functional Images,
School of Dentistry,
University of Messina,
Policlinico G. Martino
Italy

Luca Fiorillo
Department of Biomedical and
Dental Sciences, Morphological
and Functional Images,
School of Dentistry,
University of Messina,
Policlinico G. Martino
Italy

Rosa De Stefano
Department of Biomedical and
Dental Sciences, Morphological
and Functional Images,
School of Dentistry,
University of Messina,
Policlinico G. Martino
Italy

Editorial Office
MDPI
St. Alban-Anlage 66
4052 Basel, Switzerland

This is a reprint of articles from the Special Issue published online in the open access journal *Prosthesis* (ISSN 2673-1592) (available at: https://www.mdpi.com/journal/prosthesis/special_issues/ipd_prosthesis).

For citation purposes, cite each article independently as indicated on the article page online and as indicated below:

LastName, A.A.; LastName, B.B.; LastName, C.C. Article Title. *Journal Name* **Year**, *Article Number*, Page Range.

ISBN 978-3-03943-452-7 (Hbk)
ISBN 978-3-03943-453-4 (PDF)

© 2020 by the authors. Articles in this book are Open Access and distributed under the Creative Commons Attribution (CC BY) license, which allows users to download, copy and build upon published articles, as long as the author and publisher are properly credited, which ensures maximum dissemination and a wider impact of our publications.

The book as a whole is distributed by MDPI under the terms and conditions of the Creative Commons license CC BY-NC-ND.

Contents

About the Editors . . . . **vii**

Preface to "Innovative Prosthetic Device" . . . . **ix**

Luca Fiorillo, Cesare D'Amico, Anna Yurjevna Turkina, Fabiana Nicita, Giulia Amoroso and Giacomo Risitano
Endo and Exoskeleton: New Technologies on Composite Materials
Reprinted from: *Prosthesis* **2020**, 2, 1, doi:10.3390/prosthesis2010001 . . . . **1**

Luca Ortensi, Tommaso Vitali, Roberto Bonfiglioli and Francesco Grande
New Tricks in the Preparation Design for Prosthetic Ceramic Laminate Veeners
Reprinted from: *Prosthesis* **2019**, 1, 5, doi:10.3390/prosthesis1010005 . . . . **11**

Marco Portelli, Angela Militi, Antonino Logiudice and Riccardo Nucera
An Integrated Approach, Orthodontic and Prosthetic, in a Case of Maxillary Lateral Incisors Agenesis
Reprinted from: *Prosthesis* **2019**, 1, 2, doi:10.3390/prosthesis1010002 . . . . **23**

Luca Ortensi, Marco Ortensi, Andrea Minghelli and Francesco Grande
Implant-Supported Prosthetic Therapy of an Edentulous Patient: Clinical and Technical Aspects
Reprinted from: *Prosthesis* **2020**, 2, 13, doi:10.3390/prosthesis2030013 . . . . **31**

Alessandro Meduri, Rino Frisina, Miguel Rechichi and Giovanni William Oliverio
Prevalence of Meibomian Gland Dysfunction and Its Effect on Quality of Life and Ocular Discomfort in Patients with Prosthetic Eyes
Reprinted from: *Prosthesis* **2020**, 2, 10, doi:10.3390/prosthesis2020010 . . . . **45**

Helena I. Relf, Carla G. Barberio and Daniel M. Espino
A Finite Element Model for Trigger Finger
Reprinted from: *Prosthesis* **2020**, 2, 15, doi:10.3390/prosthesis2030015 . . . . **55**

Luca Fiorillo and Teresa Leanza
Worldwide 3D Printers against the New Coronavirus
Reprinted from: *Prosthesis* **2020**, 2, 9, doi:10.3390/prosthesis2020009 . . . . **73**

Leonardo Cavallo, Antonia Marcianò, Marco Cicciù and Giacomo Oteri
3D Printing beyond Dentistry during COVID 19 Epidemic: A Technical Note for Producing Connectors to Breathing Devices
Reprinted from: *Prosthesis* **2020**, 2, 5, doi:10.3390/prosthesis2020005 . . . . **77**

About the Editors

Marco Cicciù, Associate Professor. His fields of study include the technology of materials used in prostheses and implantology, biomaterials, and bone regeneration. He is the author of numerous publications in international journals and has been a speaker at many courses and conferences. He graduated in Dentistry at the University of Catania with a thesis written in collaboration with the Bioengineering Department on chewing load and stress distribution. In 2005, he obtained the title of PhD in Interceptive Orthodontics at the University of Catania and currently teaches Prosthetics and Dental Materials at the Degree Course in Dentistry of the University of Messina. In March 2017, he obtained the national scientific qualification as a full-time professor.

Luca Fiorillo, graduated with honors from the University of Messina as DDS in 2015, with a thesis entitled "Clinical differences between implants placed in native bone and implants placed in regenerated bone". In 2017, he achieved a second level master with honors in "Complex Oral Rehabilitations" at the University of Catania. Since 2018, he has been an adjunct professor at the University of Messina in the teaching of "Rehabilitative Dentistry". In 2019, he specialized in Oral Surgery at the University of Campania "Luigi Vanvitelli" in Naples. He has been a PhD student in "Bioengineering applied to Medical Sciences" at the University of Messina since 2019. In addition to authoring numerous scientific publications on oral medicine and dental materials in international, high impact journals with numerous citations, he is also an Editorial Board Member and speaker at national and international congresses.

Rosa De Stefano, graduated with honors from the University of Messina in 2014 and finished her second level master in "Psychodiagnosis and psychological evaluation" at LUMSA University of Rome in 2016. In 2019, she completed a postgraduate and higher education course entitled "The Parental Coordinator" at the University of Messina. Since 2020, she has been a subject expert in the teaching of "Psychiatry" at the University of Messina. She currently specializes in "Cognitive behavioral psychotherapy" at the Academy of Cognitive Behavioral Sciences of Calabria in Lamezia Terme. As well as being the author of numerous scientific publications on psychology, psychiatry, and oral medicine in international, high impact journals with numerous citations, she is also an Editorial Board Member and speaker at the national congress.

Preface to "Innovative Prosthetic Device"

New technologies in the biomedical field are improving the everyday lives of patients. Thanks to the advent of new biomaterials, the higher performance of materials, and the synchronization with new computer technologies, it is possible to create safer and predictable prostheses, which tend to significantly improve a patient's quality of life.

Marco Cicciù, Luca Fiorillo, Rosa De Stefano
Editors

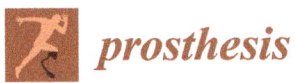

Communication

Endo and Exoskeleton: New Technologies on Composite Materials

Luca Fiorillo [1,*], Cesare D'Amico [1], Anna Yurjevna Turkina [2], Fabiana Nicita [1], Giulia Amoroso [1] and Giacomo Risitano [3]

1. Department of Biomedical and Dental Sciences and Morphological and Functional Imaging, Messina University, 98122 Messina, ME, Italy; cdamico@unime.it (C.D.); fabin92@hotmail.it (F.N.); giulia.amoroso@hotmail.it (G.A.)
2. Institute of Dentistry, Department of Therapeutic dentistry, I.M. Sechenov First Moscow State Medical University, 119146 Moscow, Russia; anna@turkin.su
3. Department of Engineering, Messina University, 98122 Messina, ME, Italy; grisitano@unime.it
* Correspondence: lfiorillo@unime.it

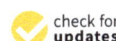

Received: 10 December 2019; Accepted: 30 December 2019; Published: 2 January 2020

Abstract: The developments in the field of rehabilitation are proceeding hand in hand with those of cybernetics, with the result of obtaining increasingly performing prostheses and rehabilitations for patients. The purpose of this work is to make a brief exposition of new technologies regarding composites materials that are used in the prosthetic and rehabilitative fields. Data collection took place on scientific databases, limited to a collection of data for the last five years, in order to present news on the innovative and actual materials. The results show that some of the most commonly used last materials are glass fibers and carbon fibers. Even in the robotics field, materials of this type are beginning to be used, thanks above all to the mechanical performances they offer. Surely these new materials, which offer characteristics similar to those in humans, could favor both the rehabilitation times of our patients, and also a better quality of life.

Keywords: biomechanical phenomena; elasticity; bioengineering; fiberglass; carbon fiber; prosthesis; rehabilitation research

---

1. Introduction

1.1. Background

In recent years new technologies in bioengineering and industrial fields have enabled the creation of new materials. These materials suitable for the rehabilitation of patients in the different districts of the body offer excellent integration capabilities and excellent biomechanical characteristics. Some of these materials also show biocompatibility characteristics, which makes them perfect to stay in contact with the body's tissues [1]. Composite materials are the materials on which the study will focus. In material science, a composite material is a heterogeneous material, that is, made up of two or more phases with different physical properties, whose properties are better than those of the phases that constitute it. Usually, the different phases in the composite are made of different materials, as in the case of carbon fiber and epoxy resin composites. However, there are exceptions where the different phases are made of the same material, such as SiC/SiC (SiC–SiC) matrix composite is a particular type of ceramic matrix composite) and self-reinforced polypropylene (SRPP) [2]. Composite materials could be both artificial or natural. Some examples of naturally occurring composite materials are wood, in which cellulose fibers are dispersed in a phase of lignin, and bones, in which collagen is reinforced by mineral apatite.

Glass fibers are used for the production of composite materials or advanced structural materials in which different components are integrated together to produce a material with superior characteristics from a physical, mechanical, chemical, aesthetic point of view. In the science and technology of materials, on the other hand, carbon fiber is a material having a thin, thread-like structure made of carbon, generally used in the production of a great variety of "composite materials", so called because they consist of two or more materials, which in this case are carbon fibers and a so-called matrix, generally of resin (or plastic or metal) whose function is to hold the resistant fibers in place (so as to maintain the correct orientation in absorbing the efforts), to protect the fibers and also to maintain the shape of the composite manufactured article. A separate discussion should be made regarding ceramic composite materials. Moreover, a different topic is all the biomaterials originating from living matter, such as bone substitutes. Thanks to new technologies, these materials, just like those under examination of the communication, could be milled or printed with CAD (Computer Aided Design) CAM (Computer Aided Manufacturing) systems [3–7]. In the technopolymers field, the composite flow molding (CFM) technology allows the production of composite materials strongly reinforced with long fiber without damaging the fibers. The reinforcement content also reaches 62% by volume to ensure maximum strength. With this process various combinations of reinforcements (carbon, glass, and Kevlar fibers) and thermoplastic resins (polyether ether ketone (PEEK), polyetherimide (PEI), polyphenylene sulfide (PPS)) are possible; the products thus obtained allow the industry to meet the growing demand for lightweight materials with excellent mechanical, chemical and thermal properties [8,9]. Form memory polymers, although already present on the market with different types of products, new materials and their development continues today to be able to identify characteristics, shapes and other possible applications. In fact their particular properties, unique in the world of plastics, mean that the still possible uses are infinite, ranging from commonly used products, made with standard industrial techniques, to functional elements of 'intelligent' junction, to pieces with good ergonomics or simply tools to improve the performance or comfort of the product in which they are inserted. In the way of "intelligent materials" there are also some membranes based on shape memory polymers. They exploit the principle of thermal vibration, that is, when the room temperature is below the activation point (dictated by the body temperature), the molecular structure stiffens, lowering the permeability, thus allowing to maintain the body temperature; when the room temperature exceeds the activation point, the molecular structure softens creating free spaces between the molecules, allowing the elimination of water vapor and excess body heat [10,11]. These membranes could be used to make water-proof and wind-resistant fabrics, which are breathable and at the same time permeable to water vapor, thus guaranteeing the anti-condensation characteristic. In the dental field, for the production of removable or fixed, implant prosthetics and orthodontic devices, the use of resins based on methacrylate (poly(methyl methacrylate) (PMMA)) and composites (bisphenol A-glycidyl methacrylate (biS-GMA)) is widespread [12]. In this manuscript, different issues related to these two technologies have been evaluated. As far as PMMA is concerned, the limits of these materials are: the imperfect repeatability of the polymerization process, limited processing times, poor biocompatibility, which could lead to the onset of considerable safety problems for the health of operators during the phases of processing of prosthetic devices, as well as of patients during the completion phases in the oral cavity and in the subsequent daily use. As for biS-GMA, the limits concern above all their operating procedures, which are quite complicated and require long transformation times; it could be associated with the high cost of the materials themselves, moreover, there are difficulties in mechanically making surfaces that are perfectly shiny and compact. This causes quite significant plaque engraftment in the oral cavity, affecting the biocompatibility of the finished devices. As for fiberglass, on the other hand, common experience shows that monolithic glass is a fragile material. If it is instead spun at diameters of less than a tenth of a millimeter it loses its characteristic fragility to become a material with high mechanical strength and resilience [12].

1.2. Aim

The aim of this manuscript is to investigate about modern and innovative prosthetic and rehabilitative materials.

2. Results

2.1. Search

The results obtained from a recent (last five years) literature search concerning innovative biomedical materials provide detailed information regarding the physical, chemical and biocompatibility characteristics of these materials; but also, their applications. Used search terms were: ("glass fiber" (All Fields) OR "carbon fiber" (All Fields) OR "composite materials" (All Fields)) AND ("Biomed J Sci Tech Res" (Journal) OR "biomedical" (All Fields)) OR ("prostheses and implants" (MeSH Terms) OR ("prostheses" (All Fields) AND "implants" (All Fields)) OR "prostheses and implants" (All Fields) OR "prosthesis" (All Fields)) OR ("rehabilitation" (MeSH Terms) OR "rehabilitation" (All Fields) OR "rehabilitative" (All Fields)).

2.2. Glass Fiber

The fragility of the common glass is due to the large number of crystallization defects that act as microfractures and stress concentration zones. On the contrary, glass fiber does not present all these defects, therefore it reaches mechanical strengths close to the theoretical resistance of the covalent bond. Different types of fibers could be distinguished according to their characteristics, which condition their use. Glass fibers are widely used in the production of structural composites in the aerospace, nautical and automotive fields, associated with different matrices, for example polyamide or epoxy, still synthetic resins [13–15]. Glass fiber is largely used in dental field, for single, multi teeth restauration (Figure 1).

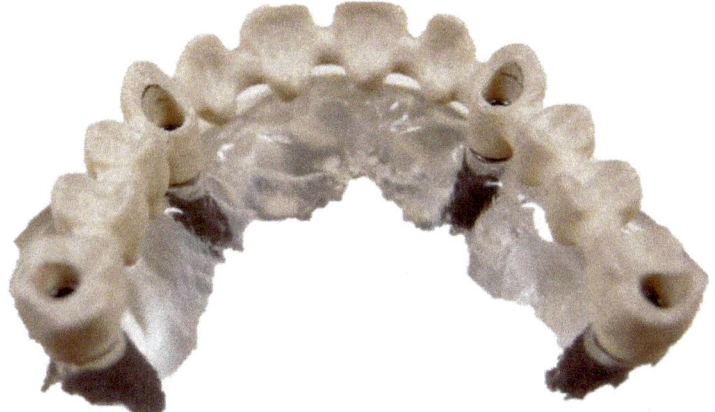

Figure 1. Glass fiber full arch implant supported dental structure. By emmekappadental.it accessed on 6 July 2019.

They are not usually used in the production of composites with metallic or ceramic matrices for which, beyond the technological problem due to the high temperature in production, it is preferred to use fibers with better performance, for example carbon fibers, in relation to the high production cost.

In the civil engineering field, glass fibers are used in the manufacture of fiber cement products. The production methods for glass fibers are:

- In disused marble, it consisted in passing the spindle through drawing nozzles;

- Disused wire rod drawing consisted of pulling glass rods to form fibers;
- With direct melting, the melt, slightly cooled but still plastic, is passed through platinum–iridium alloys (Pt-Ir) matrix, the fibers are coated with polymers to prevent them from melting together and arranged in bundles.

After spinning, the fiber is dressed to improve adhesion with the matrix to be reinforced (Table 1) [10].

Table 1. Glass fibers properties [10].

Typical Properties of Glass Fibers
Density: 2.48 g/cm^3
Elastic modulus: 90 GPa
Mechanical tensile strength (and new fiber): 4500 MPa
Percentage elongation at break: 5%

2.3. Carbon Fiber

As far as carbon fibers are concerned, these have properties similar to asbestos, but unlike the latter, their use does not entail health risks. Each weave of carbon filaments constitutes a whole formed by the union of many thousands of filaments. Each single filament has an approximately cylindrical shape with a diameter of 5–8 μm and consists almost exclusively of carbon (at least 92%). The atomic structure of the carbon fiber is similar to that of graphite, consisting of aggregates of planar-structure carbon atoms (graphene sheets) arranged according to regular hexagonal symmetry. The difference lies in the way these sheets are interconnected. Graphite is a crystalline material in which the sheets are arranged parallel to each other forming a regular structure. The chemical bonds that are established between the sheets are relatively weak, giving the graphite its characteristic delicacy and fragility. Carbon fibers have a high chemical inertness towards many aqueous solutions. They will deteriorate if they come into contact with metals and metal oxides at temperatures above 1000 K. The typical density of carbon fiber is 1750 kg/m^3. The mechanical strength of the different types of yarn varies between 2–7 GPa (Table 2) [16–20].

Table 2. Carbon Fiber commercial classification.

• GP (General Performance): characterized by lower mechanical resistance; they have a Young's modulus not exceeding 200 GPa;
• LM (Low Modulus): they have low values of the Young's modulus;
• HP (High Performance): characterized by greater mechanical strength
• HT (High Tensile Strength): they have high values of tensile strength (greater than 3000 MPa [1]) and standard values of Young's modulus (around 150–300 GPa [8])
• IM (Intermediate Modulus): have moderate values of Young's modulus (around 275–350 GPa [9])
• HM (High Modulus): they have high values of Young's modulus (greater than 300 GPa)
• UHM (UltraHigh Modulus): they have high values of Young's modulus (greater than 600 GPa).

From the point of view of the process from which they are obtained, carbon fibers are further classified into:
- Carbon fibers from polyacrylonitrile (PAN): obtained through stabilization, carbonization and possible heat treatment at high temperature of the polyacrylonitrile; 90% of carbon fibers are currently produced according to this methodology;
- Carbon fibers from isotropic pitch: obtained from pitch fibers subjected to stabilization and carbonization;

- Carbon fibers from anisotropic pitch (MPP, mesophase pitch): obtained from mesogenic pitch converted into mesophasic pitch during spinning; this mesophasic pitch is then subjected to stabilization, carbonization and high temperature heat treatment;
- Rayon carbon fibers: obtained from rayon fibers subjected to chemical pre-treatment and carbonization; this type of carbon fibers is no longer industrially produced;
- Gas phase carbon fibers: obtained from a gaseous phase containing hydrocarbons and solid catalysts; these carbon fibers are not currently marketed. Depending on the raw material used to produce the fiber, the carbon fiber could be turbostratic or graphitic, or possess a hybrid structure in which there are both turbostratic and graphitic parts. In the turbostratic carbon fiber, or with a crystalline structure formed by planes each deviated laterally with respect to the other, the sheets of carbon atoms are randomly joined or folded together. The carbon fibers obtained from the PAN are turbostratic, while the carbon fibers derived from the mesophase pitch are graphitic after heating at temperatures above 2200 °C. The turbostratic carbon fibers tend to have a greater tensile strength, while the mesophase-derived fibers subjected to heat treatment have high stiffness (Young's modulus) and high thermal conductivity [21–26].

The most commonly used method for obtaining carbon filaments is the oxidation and pyrolysis of polyacrylonitrile (PAN), a polymer obtained from the polymerization of acrylonitrile. The PAN is heated to approximately 300 °C in the presence of air, with the result of obtaining the oxidation and rupture of many hydrogen bonds established between the long polymeric chains. The oxidation product is placed in a furnace and heated to about 2000 °C in an inert gas atmosphere (for example argon), thus obtaining a radical change in the molecular structure with formation of graphite. By carrying out the heating process at the appropriate conditions, there is the condensation of the polymeric chains with the production of narrow sheets of graphene which merge and generate a single filament. The final result consists in obtaining a material with a carbon content generally ranging between 93%–95% [25].

The mechanical properties of carbon fiber could be further improved by exploiting appropriate heat treatments. Heating in the range of 1500–2000 °C results in the so-called carbonization with the formation of a material with a high tensile strength (5650 MPa), while the carbon fiber subjected to graphitization (i.e., to a heating at 2500–3000 °C) shows a higher modulus of elasticity (531 GPa). Carbon fiber is mainly used to reinforce composite materials, in particular those with a polymeric matrix. The materials thus obtained have high strength, lightness, low cost, and a certain aesthetic value. For these reasons, carbon fiber materials are widely used in a multiplicity of areas where the weight and mechanical resistance of the object are decisive factors or in consumer products simply for aesthetic purposes [26].

The lightness of these materials is also exploited in the sports field, where the lower weight of the sports equipment allows to increase the resistance of the athletes; in particular, these materials are used in the construction of:

- Racing car
- Bicycles
- Canoes
- Water skiing
- Soles of some soccer shoes
- Golf clubs
- Fishing rods
- Tennis rackets
- Archery
- Protective helmets
- Bodywork and components for rc cars
- Aircraft coverings
- Professional swimming costumes

Another area where the lightness and low cost of carbon fiber materials are exploited is the music industry [10].

Carbon fibers could also be associated with matrices in non-polymeric material. Due to the formation of carbides (for example, water-soluble aluminum carbide) and problems related to corrosion phenomena, the use of carbon in metal matrix composites is underdeveloped. Carbon–carbon (RCC, reinforced carbon–carbon) consists of a reinforcement of carbon fiber in a graphite matrix and is used in applications that require exposure to high temperatures, such as in the case of heat shields for spacecraft or brakes of Formula 1 cars. This material is also used for high temperature gas filtration, as a high surface area corrosion resistant electrode, and as an antistatic component.

Carbon fiber is increasingly used to manufacture medical equipment due to both its transparency to X-rays and its robustness. Carbon fiber could be found on:

- Tables for supporting and positioning patients in radiological rooms
- Mobility aids such as crutches [20] orthopedic or Canadian, sticks, walkers, or wheelchairs
- Orthopedic equipment such as orthoses, prostheses or exoskeletons, prosthetic heart valves (Figures 2 and 3) (Table 3) [27,28].

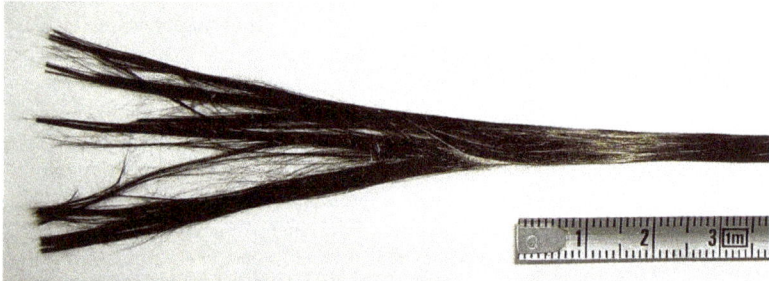

Figure 2. Carbon fiber filaments. Public Domain image.

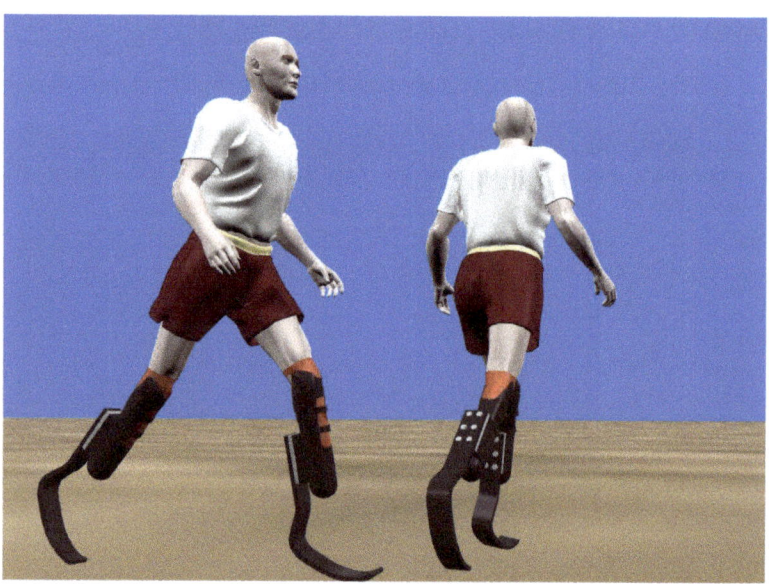

Figure 3. "Flex-Foot Cheetah" carbon prosthetic foot. By Anthony Appleyard CC BY SA 3.0.

Table 3. Carbon vs. glass fibers mechanical features [10,25].

	Glass Fibers	Carbon Fibers
Mechanical tensile strength (Pa)	1500 to 4500 MPa	150 to 600 GPa

3. Discussion

The composite fibers therefore appear to give excellent biomechanical results and their biomechanical characteristics offer performance useful for use also as an endoprosthesis. An important aspect is represented by the fact that these materials, even before they are made with printing or milling systems, could be appropriately designed in such a way that their design respects the necessary biomechanical properties. [27–29]. These simulations could be performed by discretizing a real system and performing a finite element simulation [30–32]. Glass fiber finds its primary application as a reinforcement for long-term temporary crowns, for the temporary Toronto Bridge or the Maryland bridge, and for bridges on inlays. It could be used for bridges or inlays coated with dental composite for aesthetic purposes. Its advantages are: high resistance and elasticity; biocompatibility; adhesion to composites and resins; and optimal translucency. Among the various materials used in the dental field, carbon fiber is certainly one of the most innovative and stand outs from other polymers due to its great capacity to absorb loads, offering maximum patient comfort. It is no coincidence that this material is used in the manufacture of dental prostheses that require exceptional mechanical performance, such as the Toronto Bridge or crowns on implants. In this case the carbon fiber is used as a reinforcement support and generally in most restorative methods. All this was possible also thanks to the development and improvement of adhesive techniques, which allowed an ever increasing use of polymers in the dental field. Other materials already known, such as titanium, are able to be used in contact with tissues and to build prostheses [33,34], but composite materials, as already mentioned, are able to combine the mechanical characteristics of their components [35–41]; thus, obtaining hybrid materials with unique characteristics.

4. Materials and Methods

The literature search for this Communication was carried out on the most common Scopus, Pubmed, Embase, Clarivate Analytics scientific databases. The aim was to obtain the highest possible number of results on composite materials concerning the prosthetic field. Furthermore, it was to include only innovative materials and technological and prosthetic innovations.

Author Contributions: Conceptualization, L.F.; methodology, L.F.; investigation, L.F.; data curation, L.F. and G.A.; writing—review and editing, L.F.; writing—original draft, C.D.; investigation, A.Y.T.; visualization F.N.; supervision and project administration, G.R. All authors have read and agreed to the published version of the manuscript.

Funding: This research received no external funding.

Conflicts of Interest: The authors declare no conflict of interest.

References

1. Cicciù, M. Prosthesis: New Technological Opportunities and Innovative Biomedical Devices. *Prosthesis* **2019**, *1*, 1–2. [CrossRef]
2. Katoh, Y.; Kohyama, A.; Nozawa, T.; Sato, M. SiC/SiC composites through transient eutectic-phase route for fusion applications. *J. Nucl. Mater.* **2004**, *329–333*, 587–591. [CrossRef]
3. Pizzicannella, J.; Diomede, F.; Gugliandolo, A.; Chiricosta, L.; Bramanti, P.; Merciaro, I.; Orsini, T.; Mazzon, E.; Trubiani, O. 3D Printing PLA/Gingival Stem Cells/EVs Upregulate miR-2861 and -210 during Osteoangiogenesis Commitment. *Int. J. Mol. Sci.* **2019**, *20*, 3256. [CrossRef] [PubMed]
4. Jacobs, A.; Gaulier, M.; Duval, A.; Renaudin, G. Silver Doping Mechanism in Bioceramics—From Ag+: Doped HAp to Ag°/BCP Nanocomposite. *Crystals* **2019**, *9*, 326. [CrossRef]

5. Ferracini, R.; Bistolfi, A.; Garibaldi, R.; Furfaro, V.; Battista, A.; Perale, G. Composite Xenohybrid Bovine Bone-Derived Scaffold as Bone Substitute for the Treatment of Tibial Plateau Fractures. *Appl. Sci.* **2019**, *9*, 2675. [CrossRef]
6. Chen, S.; Auriat, A.M.; Li, T.; Stumpf, T.R.; Wylie, R.; Chen, X.; Willerth, S.M.; DeRosa, M.; Tarizian, M.; Cao, X.; et al. Advancements in Canadian Biomaterials Research in Neurotraumatic Diagnosis and Therapies. *Processes* **2019**, *7*, 336. [CrossRef]
7. Ali, S.; Abdul Rani, A.M.; Mufti, R.A.; Hastuty, S.; Hussain, M.; Shehzad, N.; Baig, Z.; Abdu Aliyu, A.A. An Efficient Approach for Nitrogen Diffusion and Surface Nitriding of Boron-Titanium Modified Stainless Steel Alloy for Biomedical Applications. *Metals* **2019**, *9*, 755. [CrossRef]
8. Paryag, A.; Lowe, J.; Rafeek, R. Colored Gingiva Composite Used for the Rehabilitation of Gingiva Recessions and Non-Carious Cervical Lesions. *Dent. J.* **2017**, *5*, 33. [CrossRef]
9. Chinelatti, M.A.; Santos, E.L.; Tirapelli, C.; Pires-de-Souza, F.C.P. Effect of Methods of Biosilicate Microparticle Application on Dentin Adhesion. *Dent. J.* **2019**, *7*, 35. [CrossRef]
10. Corigliano, P.; Crupi, V.; Epasto, G.; Guglielmino, E.; Risitano, G. Fatigue Assessment by Thermal Analysis during Tensile Tests on Steel. *Procedia Eng.* **2015**, *109*, 210–218. [CrossRef]
11. Cucinotta, F.; Guglielmino, E.; Risitano, G.; Sfravara, F. Assessment of Damage Evolution in Sandwich Composite Material Subjected to Repeated Impacts by Means Optical Measurements. *Procedia Struct. Integr.* **2016**, *2*, 3660–3667. [CrossRef]
12. Giudice, G.; Cicciù, M.; Cervino, G.; Lizio, A.; Visco, A. Flowable resin and marginal gap on tooth third medial cavity involving enamel and radicular cementum: A SEM evaluation of two restoration techniques. *Indian J. Dent. Res.* **2012**, *23*, 763–769. [PubMed]
13. Taheri, H.; Hassen, A.A. Nondestructive Ultrasonic Inspection of Composite Materials: A Comparative Advantage of Phased Array Ultrasonic. *Appl. Sci.* **2019**, *9*, 1628. [CrossRef]
14. Spelter, A.; Bergmann, S.; Bielak, J.; Hegger, J. Long-Term Durability of Carbon-Reinforced Concrete: An Overview and Experimental Investigations. *Appl. Sci.* **2019**, *9*, 1651. [CrossRef]
15. Gao, K.; Li, Z.; Zhang, J.; Tu, J.; Li, X. Experimental Research on Bond Behavior between GFRP Bars and Stirrups-Confined Concrete. *Appl. Sci.* **2019**, *9*, 1340. [CrossRef]
16. Zhou, W.; Zhang, P.-f.; Zhang, Y.-n. Acoustic Emission Based on Cluster and Sentry Function to Monitor Tensile Progressive Damage of Carbon Fiber Woven Composites. *Appl. Sci.* **2018**, *8*, 2265. [CrossRef]
17. Zhao, Q.; Zhang, K.; Zhu, S.; Xu, H.; Cao, D.; Zhao, L.; Zhang, R.; Yin, W. Review on the Electrical Resistance/Conductivity of Carbon Fiber Reinforced Polymer. *Appl. Sci.* **2019**, *9*, 2390. [CrossRef]
18. Otani, T.; Hashimoto, K.; Miyamae, S.; Ueta, H.; Natsuhara, A.; Sakaguchi, M.; Kawakami, Y.; Lim, H.-O.; Takanishi, A. Upper-Body Control and Mechanism of Humanoids to Compensate for Angular Momentum in the Yaw Direction Based on Human Running. *Appl. Sci.* **2018**, *8*, 44. [CrossRef]
19. Kim, R.-W.; Kim, C.-M.; Hwang, K.-H.; Kim, S.-R. Embedded Based Real-Time Monitoring in the High-Pressure Resin Transfer Molding Process for CFRP. *Appl. Sci.* **2019**, *9*, 1795. [CrossRef]
20. Ayyagari, S.; Al-Haik, M. Enhancing the Viscoelastic Performance of Carbon Fiber Composites by Incorporating CNTs and ZnO Nanofillers. *Appl. Sci.* **2019**, *9*, 2281. [CrossRef]
21. Vercio, R.C.; Basmajian, H.G. Fracture of a Carbon Fiber Reinforced Intramedullary Femoral Nail. *J. Am. Acad. Orthop. Surg.* **2019**, *27*, e585–e588. [CrossRef] [PubMed]
22. Pesce, P.; Lagazzo, A.; Barberis, F.; Repetto, L.; Pera, F.; Baldi, D.; Menini, M. Mechanical characterisation of multi vs. uni-directional carbon fiber frameworks for dental implant applications. *Mater. Sci. Eng. C Mater. Biol. Appl.* **2019**, *102*, 186–191. [CrossRef] [PubMed]
23. Mehl, B.T.; Martin, R.S. Integrating 3D Cell Culture of PC12 Cells with Microchip-Based Electrochemical Detection. *Anal. Methods Adv. Methods Appl.* **2019**, *11*, 1064–1072. [CrossRef] [PubMed]
24. Liu, H.; Zhang, S.; Yang, J.; Ji, M.; Yu, J.; Wang, M.; Chai, X.; Yang, B.; Zhu, C.; Xu, J. Preparation, Stabilization and Carbonization of a Novel Polyacrylonitrile-Based Carbon Fiber Precursor. *Polymers* **2019**, *11*, 1150. [CrossRef]
25. Gao, Y.; Duan, X.; Jiang, P.; Zhang, H.; Liu, J.; Wen, S.; Zhao, X.; Zhang, L. Molecular dynamics simulation of the electrical conductive network formation of polymer nanocomposites by utilizing diblock copolymer-mediated nanoparticles. *Soft Matter* **2019**, *15*. [CrossRef]
26. Erdenechimeg, K.; Jeong, H.I.; Lee, C.M. A Study on the Laser-Assisted Machining of Carbon Fiber Reinforced Silicon Carbide. *Materials* **2019**, *12*, 2061. [CrossRef]

27. Risitano, A.; Clienti, C.; Risitano, G. Determination of fatigue limit by mono-axial tensile specimens using thermal analysis. *Key Eng. Mater.* **2009**, *452*, 361–364. [CrossRef]
28. Fargione, G.; Tringale, D.; Guglielmino, E.; Risitano, G. Fatigue characterization of mechanical components in service. *Frattura ed Integrita Strutturale* **2013**, *26*, 143–155. [CrossRef]
29. Cicciù, M.; Cervino, G.; Milone, D.; Risitano, G. FEM investigation of the stress distribution over mandibular bone due to screwed overdenture positioned on dental implants. *Materials* **2018**, *11*, 1512. [CrossRef]
30. Bramanti, E.; Cervino, G.; Lauritano, F.; Fiorillo, L.; D'Amico, C.; Sambataro, S.; Denaro, D.; Fama, F.; Ierardo, G.; Polimeni, A.; et al. FEM and Von Mises Analysis on Prosthetic Crowns Structural Elements: Evaluation of Different Applied Materials. *Sci. World J.* **2017**, *2017*, 1029574. [CrossRef]
31. Cervino, G.; Romeo, U.; Lauritano, F.; Bramanti, E.; Fiorillo, L.; D'Amico, C.; Milone, D.; Laino, L.; Campolongo, F.; Rapisarda, S.; et al. Fem and Von Mises Analysis of OSSTEM (r) Dental Implant Structural Components: Evaluation of Different Direction Dynamic Loads. *Open Dent. J.* **2018**, *12*, 219–229. [CrossRef] [PubMed]
32. Portelli, M.; Militi, A.; Logiudice, A.; Nucera, R. An Integrated Approach, Orthodontic and Prosthetic, in a Case of Maxillary Lateral Incisors Agenesis. *Prosthesis* **2020**, *1*, 3–10. [CrossRef]
33. McGrory, A.; McGrory, B.; Rana, A.; Babikian, G. Incidence of Heterotopic Ossification in Anterior Based Muscle Sparing Total Hip Arthroplasty: A Retrospective Radiographic Review. *Prosthesis* **2020**, *1*, 11–15. [CrossRef]
34. Frossard, L.; Jones, M.; Stewart, I.; Leggat, P.; Schuetz, M.; Langton, C. Kinetics of Lower Limb Prosthesis: Automated Detection of Vertical Loading Rate. *Prosthesis* **2020**, *1*, 16–28. [CrossRef]
35. Ortensi, L.; Vitali, T.; Bonfiglioli, R.; Grande, F. New Tricks in the Preparation Design for Prosthetic Ceramic Laminate Veeners. *Prosthesis* **2020**, *1*, 29–40. [CrossRef]
36. Cicciù, M.; Cervino, G.; Terranova, A.; Risitano, G.; Raffaele, M.; Cucinotta, F.; Santonocito, D.; Fiorillo, L. Prosthetic and Mechanical Parameters of the Facial Bone under the Load of Different Dental Implant Shapes: A Parametric Study. *Prosthesis* **2020**, *1*, 41–53. [CrossRef]
37. Cervino, G.; Montanari, M.; Santonocito, D.; Nicita, F.; Baldari, R.; De Angelis, C.; Storni, G.; Fiorillo, L. Comparison of Two Low-Profile Prosthetic Retention System Interfaces: Preliminary Data of an In Vitro Study. *Prosthesis* **2020**, *1*, 54–60. [CrossRef]
38. Iovino, P.; Di Sarno, A.; De Caro, V.; Mazzei, C.; Santonicola, A.; Bruno, V. Screwdriver Aspiration During Oral Procedures: A Lesson for Dentists and Gastroenterologists. *Prosthesis* **2020**, *1*, 61–68. [CrossRef]
39. Sambataro, S.; Cervino, G.; Fiorillo, L.; Cicciu, M. Upper First Premolar Positioning Evaluation for the Stability of the Dental Occlusion: Anatomical Considerations. *J. Craniofac. Surg.* **2018**, *29*, 1366–1369. [CrossRef]
40. Cicciu, M.; Fiorillo, L.; Herford, A.S.; Crimi, S.; Bianchi, A.; D'Amico, C.; Laino, L.; Cervino, G. Bioactive Titanium Surfaces: Interactions of Eukaryotic and Prokaryotic Cells of Nano Devices Applied to Dental Practice. *Biomedicines* **2019**, *7*, 12. [CrossRef]
41. Cervino, G.; Fiorillo, L.; Iannello, G.; Santonocito, D.; Risitano, G.; Cicciù, M. Sandblasted and Acid Etched Titanium Dental Implant Surfaces Systematic Review and Confocal Microscopy Evaluation. *Materials* **2019**, *12*, 1763. [CrossRef] [PubMed]

 © 2020 by the authors. Licensee MDPI, Basel, Switzerland. This article is an open access article distributed under the terms and conditions of the Creative Commons Attribution (CC BY) license (http://creativecommons.org/licenses/by/4.0/).

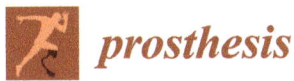

Case Report

New Tricks in the Preparation Design for Prosthetic Ceramic Laminate Veeners

Luca Ortensi [1],*, Tommaso Vitali [2], Roberto Bonfiglioli [3] and Francesco Grande [4]

1. Department of Prosthodontics, University of Catania, 95123 Catania, Italy
2. Private Practice, Castiglione del Lago, 06061 Perugia, Italy; tommaso.vitali83@gmail.com
3. Private Practice, 40100 Bologna, Italy; roberto.bonfiglioli@c-oralia.it
4. Department of Oral Surgery, University of Bologna, 40132 Bologna, Italy; francesco.grande6@unibo.it
* Correspondence: luca@ortensistrocchi.it; Tel.: +39-051-221-916

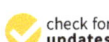

Received: 12 October 2019; Accepted: 27 October 2019; Published: 30 October 2019

Abstract: Background: The prosthetic preparation of the teeth for ceramic laminate veneers has to follow the minimally invasive concept brought by the modern Conservative Dentistry and Prosthodontics. However, during the cementation phase under the rubber dam, the loss of the esthetics landmarks could lead to errors in the future positioning of the laminate veneers. Methods: In this article the authors show an accurate operative prosthetic protocol using different fine intraoperative maneuvers and tricks for the realization of ceramic laminates in order to solve the problems of the cementation phase. Results: The treatment of the anterior sector of the upper maxilla with porcelain laminate veneers was realized in a 30 years old woman with aesthetic issues. Conclusion: Different fine intraoperative maneuvers and tricks during teeth preparation, master impression and rubber dam positioning could reduce errors occurring in the cementation phase and increase the predictability of the results.

Keywords: ceramic laminate veneers; teeth preparation; dental esthetics; dental porcelain; rubber dam; prosthetic treatment planning; Digital Smile System

1. Introduction

The advent of adhesive restorative materials has introduced minimal intervention principles in restorative dentistry and prosthodontics [1]. The necessity of making undercuts in the dental tissue has been abandoned due to new adhesive techniques that allow for the reconstruction of the cavities without excessive preparation for macromechanical retention [2]. Also, the correct use of ceramic and composite materials with rigorous adhesive procedures allows a sound tissue preservation because of the minimally or even noninvasive (additive) approach, which is innovative, highly esthetic, and predictable in terms of both result and long-term prognosis [3,4]. The aesthetics have also improved because of the high level of biomimetics of these new adhesive materials, which also allow for a better function within the oral cavity. Because of the hydrophobic characteristics of these materials, the correct use of adhesive techniques requires an effective moisture control in order to promote the bonding of the restorative materials and then to reduce failure rates of dental restorative treatments [5]. Therefore, a performing isolation system that creates a barrier from the rest of the person's mouth is necessary before executing adhesive procedures in order to control the moisture and microbes. Using a rubber dam can isolate the teeth and this allows the teeth to be restored dry and with relatively less exposure to intraoral bacteria [6]. Other advantages of the use of a rubber dam include superior isolation of the tooth to be treated from the saliva in the mouth [7], improved visibility, reduced mirror fogging, enhanced visual contrast, soft tissue retraction [8], protection of the person by preventing ingestion or aspiration of instruments, materials [9] and preventing oral soft tissues from contact with harmful materials used during operative procedures, such as phosphoric acids [10].

However, some problems related to the use of the rubber dam could be faced during prosthetic treatments, especially when rehabilitation of the anterior regions of the oral cavity has to be done with different indirect aesthetic restorations such as composite or ceramic laminate veneers (lithium disilicate, feldspathic ceramics). Incorrect rubber dam clamps placement may occupy a space that is needed for the restoration, besides possible damages to the marginal gingiva around the teeth. In addition, the use of the rubber dam leads to a loss of esthetics landmarks such as the midsagittal line, with subsequent difficulties [11] for the correct placement of the veneers on the teeth. The small holes made in the sheet could disagree with the position of the teeth that have to be treated. In addition, inaccuracy in the reproduction of the position of the interdental contact points in the gypsum model during indirect restorations could lead to errors in the future positioning of the laminate veneers. The aim of this article is to present a clinical case report demonstrating an accurate operative protocol using different fine intraoperative maneuvers and tricks for the realization of prosthetic ceramic laminates in order to solve the problems mentioned above.

2. Materials and Methods

A 30 years old woman presented at our attention with aesthetic issues. She expressed the desire to change her smile because her anterior maxillary teeth seemed small and disharmonious because of the discrepancy in the dimension between each other. She refused to undergo orthodontic treatment for her situation of malocclusion (she presented) but she was very motivated for obtaining a more acceptable smile.

Clinical examination showed a right posterior crossbite with a normal overbite and overjet, superior and inferior dental midline misalignment and Altered Passive Eruption (APE) of 2.1 and 2.2. Radiographic evaluation showed an absence of endodontic and periodontal lesions. Esthetic analysis highlighted an important gummy smile, superior and inferior dental midline misalignment, gingival ogives asymmetry. The patient showed good oral hygiene habits. Then, in light of the anamnesis, objective and radiographic examinations, chief complaint, the treatment of the anterior sector of the upper maxilla with porcelain laminate veneers was proposed.

The operative sequence is structured as follows:

1. Intra- and extraoral esthetic analysis of the patient, with static photographic pre-prosthetic documentation.
2. Digital previsualization by means of DSS (digital smile system) and patient's approval of the digital prosthetic previsualization.
3. Clinical previsualization by means of a mock-up or aesthetic pre-evaluative temporaries (APTs), based on a virtual wax-up.
4. Evaluation and treatment of endodontic, mucogingival, and/or orthodontic problems, where necessary.
5. Preparation of the teeth added by the mock-up with proper modifications of the regular technique.
6. Master impression with adaptations.
7. Manufacturing of prosthetic ceramic laminate veneers (feldspathic or lithium disilicate).
8. Try-in and adhesive cementation under rubber dam isolation by using new different tricks.

2.1. Treatment Planning and Realization

In the first objective clinical examination of the patient, a correct diagnosis, including medical and dental history, dental and periodontal screening with periodontal probing depths recording, full mouth intraoral X-rays set and initial clinical intraoral and extraoral photos was done (Figures 1 and 2).

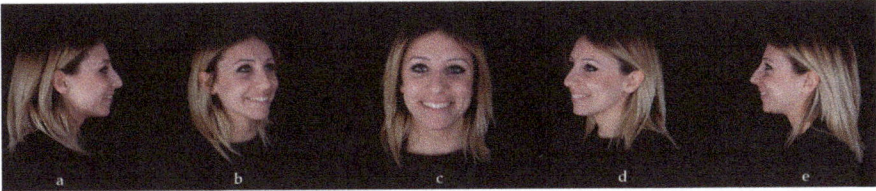

Figure 1. Extraoral facial photos: (**a**) right lateral view; (**b**) three quarter right view; (**c**) frontal view; (**d**) three quarter left view; (**e**) left lateral view.

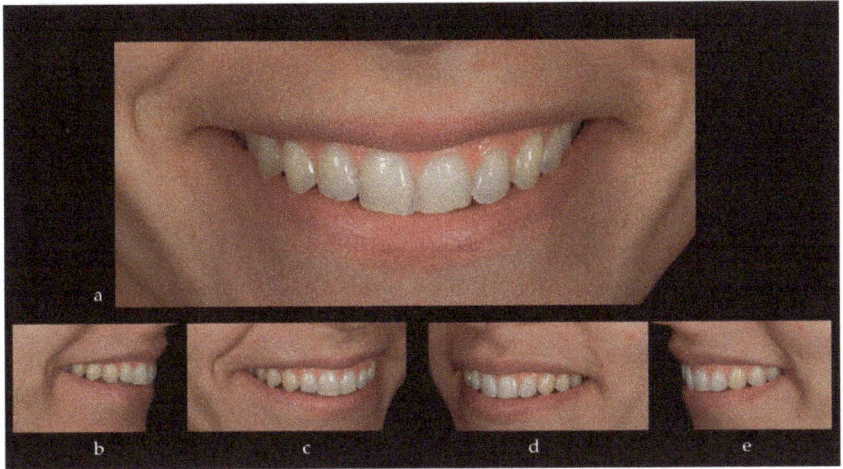

Figure 2. Extraoral photos of the smile: (**a**) frontal view; (**b**) right lateral view; (**c**) three quarter right view; (**d**) three quarter left view; (**e**) left lateral view.

A preliminary phase with oral professional hygiene and full mouth disinfection was performed to achieve the health oral conditions necessary to do a correct treatment planning.

Oral impressions with alginate material (Hydrogum 5, Zhermack) have been taken and also digital oral impressions were detected for comparison.

Then a treatment proposal with digital prosthodontic previsualization was shown to the patient with the aid of the Digital Smile System. Longer teeth with more harmonic shapes in the cervical and incisal portions were digitally projected and the patients was informed about all the next steps of the treatment (Figure 3).

After patient approval of the previsualization, the treatment starts by performing a mucogingival surgery with the aid of a mockup used as an oral surgical guide for a highly accurate definition of the emergency profiles and gingival parabolas (Figure 4). A multiple coronal flap technique was used and the gingiva excesses were cut. Little osteotomy and osteoplasty were done in order to reach the accurate vertical dimensions of the teeth established during the treatment planning. In this manner we were able to assess the correct biological width in real-time by placing the mock-up on the teeth. The epithelium of the anatomical papillae was removed and absorbable sutures were applied.

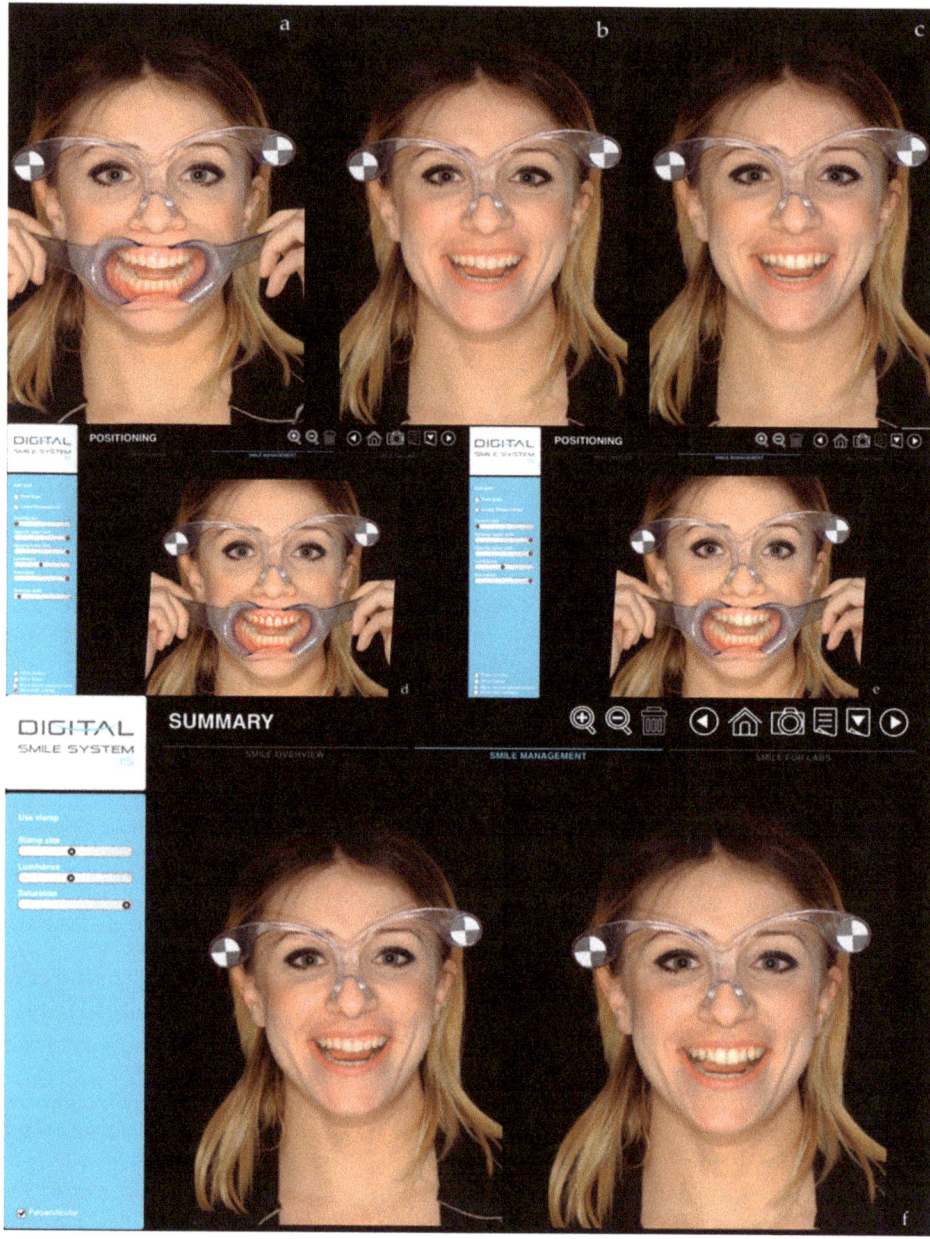

Figure 3. Digital planning with DSS (digital smile system): (**a**) photo with cheek retractors and DSS glasses during mouth opening; (**b**) photo with full smile and DSS glasses; (**c**) virtual digital project; (**d**) DSS software screen with design outline and final project; (**e**) DSS software screen with final project; (**f**) comparison between initial clinical photo and final virtual project.

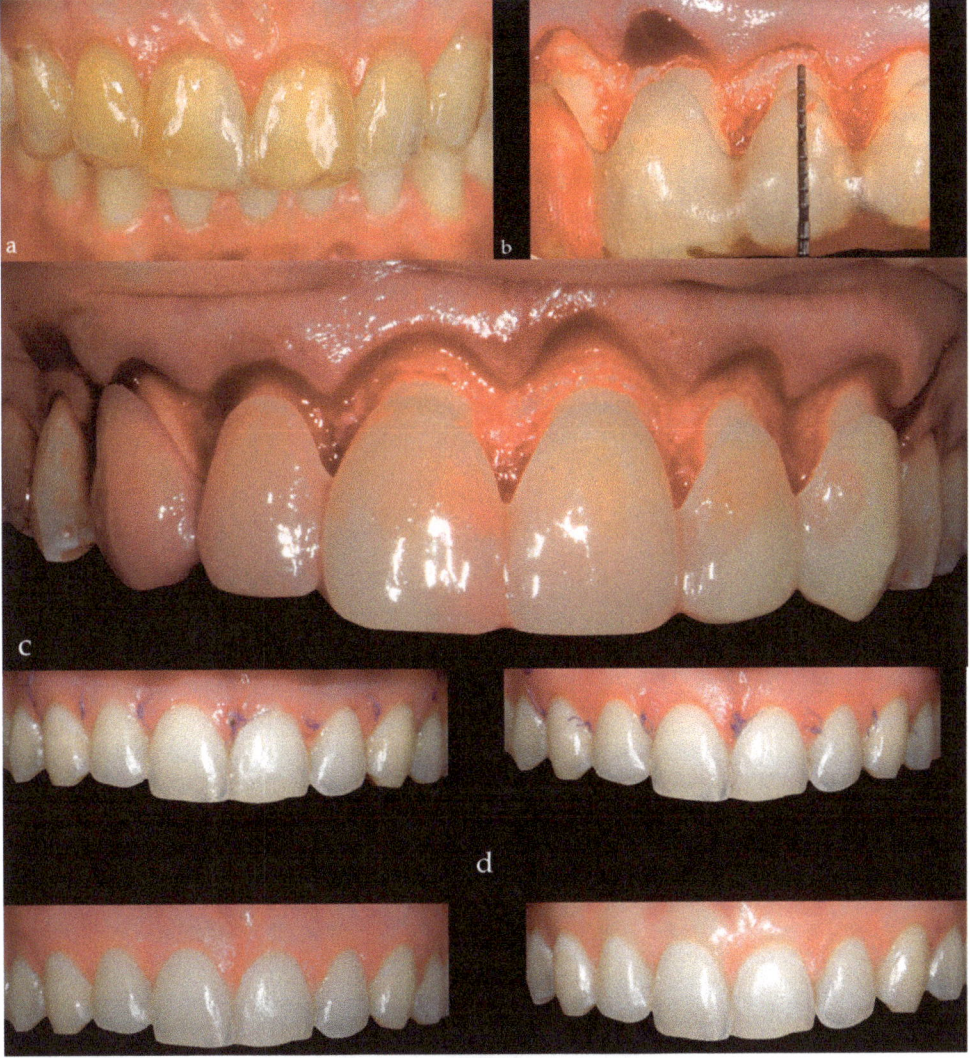

Figure 4. Periodontal surgery phases: (**a**) mock-up/periodontal surgical guide; (**b**) biologic width check with surgical guide; (**c**) biologic width check with mock-up; (**d**) follow-up (1–6 weeks postop).

After a healing period of 12 months, as suggested by Pontoriero and Carnevale [12], prosthetic phase with preparation of teeth 1.3, 1.2, 1.1, 2.1, 2.2 and 2.3 for porcelain laminate veneers was done. Then a resin mock-up (C&B, A3.5, NextDent B.V.) was applied on the teeth elected for veneer preparations (Figure 5).

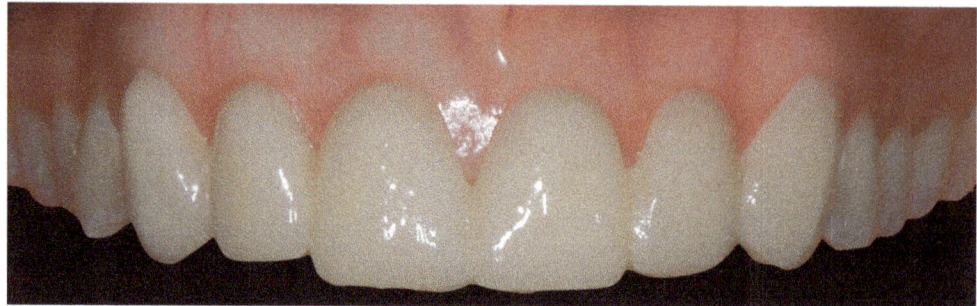

Figure 5. Resin mock-up on teeth elected for veeners.

After trying the mock-up from the esthetically and mechanically point of view, a minimal iuxta-gingival butt joint preparation was done. A reduction of 0.5 mm of the buccal plate and of 1.5 mm of the incisal portion of the teeth added by the mock-up [13] was performed (Figure 6). Teeth 1.3, 1.2, 1.1, 2.1, 2.2 and 2.3 were prepared.

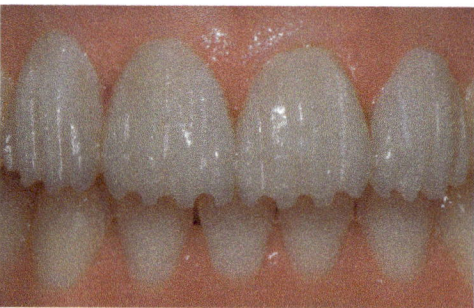

Figure 6. Preparation of the teeth added by the mock-up with proper modifications of the regular technique.

After the buccal plate preparation, a little hole made by a round bur at the center of each tooth was realized in order to ensure the correct positioning of the prosthetic veneers during the cementation phase under rubber dam (Figure 7).

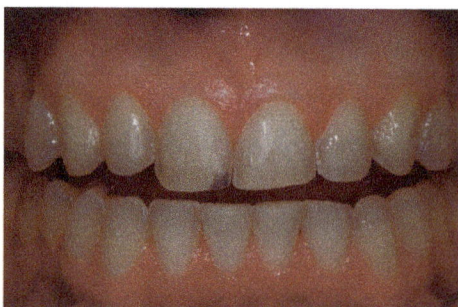

Figure 7. Teeth 1.3, 1.2, 1.1, 2.1, 2.2 and 2.3 prepared. Clinical aspects of dental preparations.

A stock tray was chosen to take the master impression, considering that around undercuts, the distance of the tooth to the try wall needs to be at least twice the depth of the undercut [14]. Application of VPS adhesive on the tray and subsequent drying were done. For an accurate reproduction of the margin preparation, two retraction cords—the first smaller and the second bigger—were positioned around the prepared teeth according to the double cord retraction technique [15].

In order to facilitate the technician in his work, seven small metal sectional matrixes were sprinkled with VPS adhesive and fixed between the anterior teeth and between canines and first premolars before taking the oral impression (Figure 8).

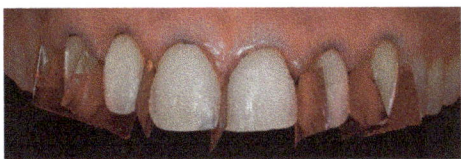

Figure 8. Metal sectional matrixes between teeth before vinyl-polysiloxane master impression.

Then, a master impression with a one-step technique using vinyl-polysiloxane impression materials (Acquasil Ultra mono e XLV regular set Dentsply) was taken.

The mockup realized in the first prosthetic phase was used again for making temporary veneers, which were attached on the teeth by using the spot-etching technique (Figure 9).

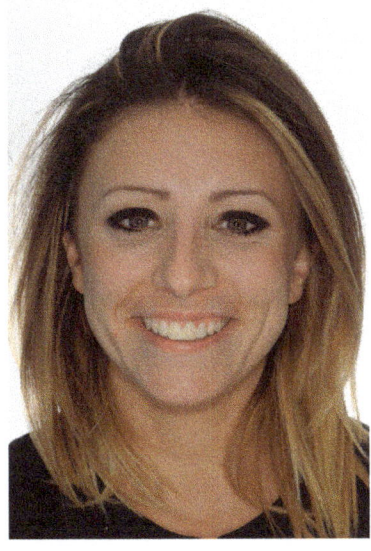

Figure 9. Mock-up for temporary veneers attached by spot-etching technique.

2.2. Cementation Phase

Six lithium disilicate veneer restorations were manufactured by the technician after seven days from the master impression (Figures 10 and 11).

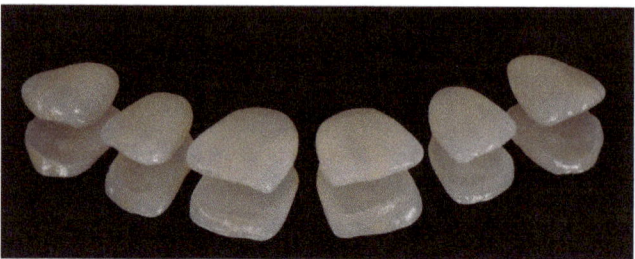

Figure 10. Lithium disilicate veneers.

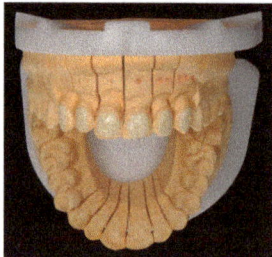

Figure 11. Master model.

The following prosthetic clinical steps for the cementation phase were:

- Removal of the temporary restorations and polishing of the tooth surfaces in order to remove the provisional cement.
- Definitive restorations try-in on prepared teeth by using a water-soluble cement (Relyx Try-in paste 3M). Each single veneer was prosthetically evaluated for proximal contacts, shade match, contour, and marginal adaptation. After that evaluation, the definitive cementation phase could follow. Otherwise little reshaping of the veneer could be done if the ceramic permits those modifications or taking other oral impression. In this phase we could also try different colored translucent cements in order to visualize the resulting effect on the color and establishing color and viscosity of the cement of choice.
- Triple zero retraction cord positioning around prepared teeth (1.3, 1.2, 1.1, 2.1, 2.2 and 2.3).
- Rubber dam isolation from 1.5 to 2.5 with n°2 clamps and correct retraction in the apical part of the teeth by using an interdental floss ligature for each tooth for obtaining a correct moisture control.
- Sandblasting with aluminum oxide particles of the prepared teeth surfaces in order to enhance the bond strength [16].
- Positioning of the modified n°9 clamp modified on the first tooth for cementation. This modification allows the correct positioning of the veneer without any interferences between the most apical point of the veneer (zenith of the veneer) and the clamp beaks (Figure 12).

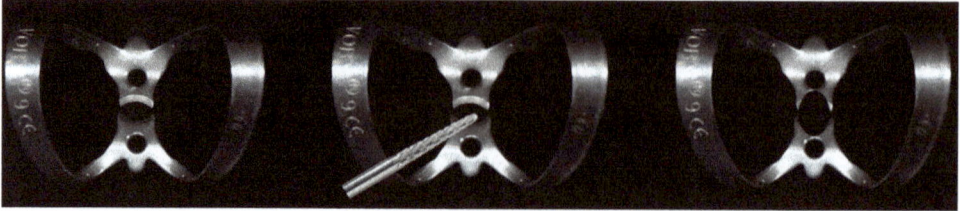

Figure 12. N°9 modified clamp.

In order to reach a better control of the interdental contact point, the prosthetic cementation has begun from one central incisor and then continued alternating the tooth for cementation;

- Teflon application on adjacent teeth or matrix positioning in order to avoid contamination of the other elements (Figure 13);
- Etching of the tooth surface prepared with 37% orthophosphoric acid. Subsequent rinsing, drying and application of bonding agent.
- Etching with 9.5 hydrofluoric acid for 20 seconds and cleaning of the internal surface of lithium disilicate veneers [17].
- Application of the universal bond, which contains silane on the internal surface of the lithium disilicate veneers (or silane and bonding applied in two different subsequent steps) [18];
- Elimination of the bonding excesses and drying of the surface of the application in order to evaporate its volatile component.
- Light curing of the adhesive on tooth and veneer surfaces.
- Positioning of the veneer on tooth surface with Relyx veneer (3M) cement and removal of the cement excesses prior to photopolymerization.
- Repetition of the procedure for each tooth prepared prior to controlling the interdental contact points.
- Removal of the rubber dam.
- Removal of the other excesses of bonding agent and cement in order to obtain more regular contours.
- Control of the occlusal and interdental contacts (Figures 14 and 15).

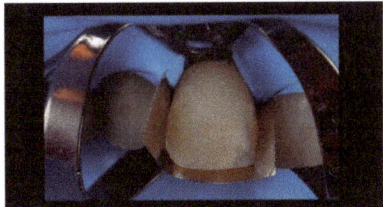

Figure 13. Matrix application on adjacent teeth positioning during cementation phase.

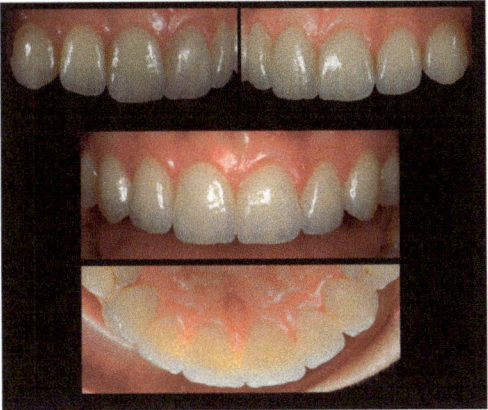

Figure 14. Post cementation check.

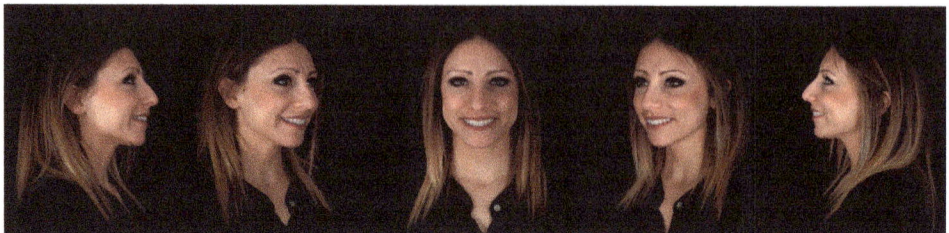

Figure 15. Extraoral final photos: teeth reharmonization.

3. Discussion

The rehabilitation of the anterior sector is always a challenging procedure for the prosthodontist. This is especially true when young patients with high aesthetic requests are involved in the prosthetic treatment.

According to Magne and Belser [19], ceramic laminate veneers represent a well-documented, effective, and predictable treatment option when teeth bleaching was ineffective and when major morphologic modifications and extensive restorations in adult patients are required.

The prosthetic preparation of the teeth for ceramic laminate veneers has to follow the minimally invasive concept brought by the modern Prosthodontic and Conservative Dentistry in order to provide esthetic and functional rehabilitation. Three different preparation designs have been suggested regarding the incisal edge preparation: the feathered incisal edge, the butt joint and the overlapped incisal edge with palatal chamfer. Some authors have found that the butt joint is the preparation that least affects the strength of the tooth and that the chamfer preparation type is more susceptible to ceramic fractures [20].

For labial surface preparation, which is the most esthetic portion of ceramic laminate veneers, an accurate preparation depth can be achieved via several methods: freehand, use of depth cuts/grooves and use of a silicon putty index obtained after the wax up or the provisional have all shown good predictable results in reducing the buccal plate for the thickness previously planned [21].

For interproximal extension, no conclusive evidence demonstrates what is the best technique to prepare. Then, the clinician has to choose for each case if it is better to not prepare or to prepare until the interproximal contact point or to slightly open the interproximal contact.

However, in some cases no teeth preparation is required to restore the teeth ("no prep technique") [22].

All these preparation techniques are based on the need to give optimal biomechanics and aesthetic characteristics—at the same time respecting the highly conservative concepts. However, in order to achieve those final goals, it is also mandatory that the prosthetic cementation phase is free of mistakes. These techniques do not consider the difficulty in maintaining the correct spatial orientation during the cementation phase, and the subsequent possibility to design a preparation for laminates in order to position in a correct way the veneers on the teeth. In this direction, we perform some different fine intraoperative maneuvers and tricks that help the clinician in the preparation of the teeth and in the subsequent placement of the laminates on the teeth prepared under the rubber dam.

The modification of the labial preparation by performing a little hole with a round bur at the center of buccal plate of the tooth is important to achieve the correct placement of the veneers under the rubber dam when extraoral and intraoral landmarks disappear. Moreover, during the prosthetic cementation phase, the attention of the clinician is mainly referred to factors such as the cement excesses and the pressure applied on the veneers during its positioning, as these factors could lead to cement the veneers in an incorrect position [23].

Another little trick that could prevent possible errors during the luting phase is the modification of number 9 hook. The objective is to avoid small shifts during veneer positioning because of the interference between the hook and the most coronal part (zenith) of the veneer itself. This adaptation consists in the elimination of the flattened part of the labial clamp beak in order to put the hook in an apical position that cannot interfere with the zenith of the veneer.

The correct positioning of the prosthetic veneers on teeth is also dependent on how accurate the technician works and how precise the fitting of the veneers is. Then, in order to facilitate the technician, during the master impression phase seven small metal sectional matrixes were sprinkled with vinyl-polysiloxane adhesive and fixed between the anterior teeth and between canines and first premolars before taking the oral impression. The goal is to highlight the interdental contact points in the model, aiding the technician to separate the teeth from each other with the bur, without any risk to remove the contact points because of the additional space obtained during the manufacturing of the cast with the removable abutments.

4. Conclusions

Adhesive and minimally invasive dentistry is nowadays a consolidated reality in Prosthetic Dentistry. New materials and techniques must guarantee a good predictability of the final goal from the beginning to the end of treatment and not only an optimal aesthetics, which could also improve.

However, other studies with more patients and longer follow-ups are required to prove the reliability of this new tricks and techniques improving the technical procedures of the treatment.

Author Contributions: Conceptualization, L.O., T.V. and F.G.; methodology, L.O., T.V and T.V.; software, L.O., T.V. and T.V.; resources, T.V.; data curation, F.G.; writing—original draft preparation, F.G.; writing—review and editing, L.O., T.V. and F.G.; visualization, L.O., T.V. and F.G.; supervision, T.V. R.B. fabricated the laminate veneers.

Funding: This research received no external funding

Acknowledgments: The authors thank Gianni Ortensi, CDT and Marco Ortensi, CDT, who fabricated the mock-up and supported laboratory digital processes.

Conflicts of Interest: The authors declare no conflict of interest.

References

1. Cicciù, M. Prosthes: New Technological Opportunities and Innovative Biomedical Devices. *Prosthesis* **2019**, *1*, 1–2. [CrossRef]
2. Mackenzie, L.; Banerjee, A. Minimally invasive direct restorations: A practical guide. *Br. Dent. J.* **2017**, *11*, 163–171. [CrossRef] [PubMed]
3. Staehle, H.J.; Wolff, D.; Frese, C. More conservative dentistry: Clinical long-term results of direct composite resin restorations. *Quintessence Int.* **2015**, *46*, 373–380.
4. Edelhoff, D.; Prandtner, O.; Saeidi Pour, R.; Liebermann, A.; Stimmelmayr, M.; Guth, J.F. Anterior restorations: The performance of ceramic veneers. *Quintessence Int.* **2018**, *49*, 89–101. [PubMed]
5. Pereira, J.R.; Pamato, S.; Vargas, M.; Junior, N.F. State of the Art of Dental Adhesive Systems. *Curr. Drug Deliv.* **2018**, *15*, 610–619. [CrossRef]
6. Wang, Y.; Li, C.; Yuan, H.; Wong, M.C.; Zou, J.; Shi, z.; Zhou, X. Rubber dam isolation for restorative treatment in dental patients. *Cochrane Database Syst. Rev.* **2016**, *9*, CD009858. [CrossRef]
7. Cochran, M.A.; Miller, C.H.; Sheldrake, M.A. The efficacy of the rubber dam as a barrier to the spread of microorganisms during dental treatment. *J. Am. Dent. Assoc.* **1989**, *119*, 141–144. [CrossRef]
8. Reid, J.S.; Callis, P.D.; Patterson, C.J.W. *Rubber Dam in Clinical Practice*, 1st ed.; Quintessence Publishing: London, UK, 1991.
9. Tiwana, K.K.; Morton, T.; Tiwana, P.S. Aspiration and ingestion in dental practice: A 10-year institutional review. *J. Am. Dent. Assoc.* **2004**, *135*, 1287–1291. [CrossRef]
10. Lynch, C.D.; McConnell, R.J. The use of micro abrasion to remove discolored enamel: A clinical report. *J. Prosthet. Dent.* **2003**, *90*, 417–419. [CrossRef]
11. Mizrahi, B. Porcelain veneers: Techniques and precautions. *Int. Dent.* **2007**, *9*, 1–4.
12. Pontoriero, R.; Carnevale, G. Surgical crown lengthening: A 12-month clinical wound healing study. *J. Periodontol.* **2001**, *72*, 841–848. [CrossRef] [PubMed]

13. Magne, P.; Magne, M. Use of additive wax up and direct intraoral mock-up for enamel preservation with porcelain laminate veneers. *Eur. J. Esthet. Dent.* **2006**, *1*, 10–19. [PubMed]
14. Millstein, P.; Maya, A.; Segura, C. Determining the accuracy of stock and custom tray impression/casts. *J. Oral Rehabil.* **1998**, *25*, 645–648. [CrossRef] [PubMed]
15. Cloyd, S.; Puri, S. Using the double-cord packing technique of tissue retraction for making crown impressions. *Dent. Today* **1999**, *18*, 54–59. [PubMed]
16. Consani, R.L.; Richter, M.M.; Mesquita, M.F.; Sinhoreti, M.A.; Guiraldo, R.D. Effect of aluminum oxide particle sandblasting on the artificial tooth-resin bond. *J. Investig. Clin. Dent.* **2010**, *1*, 144–150. [CrossRef] [PubMed]
17. Zogheib, L.V.; Bona, A.D.; Kimpara, E.T.; McCabe, J.F. Effect of hydrofluoric acid etching duration on the roughness and flexural strength of a lithium disilicate-based glass ceramic. *Braz. Dent. J.* **2011**, *22*, 45–50. [CrossRef] [PubMed]
18. Johnson, G.H.; Lepe, X.; Patterson, A.; Sch√§fer, O. Simplified cementation of lithium disilicate crowns: Retention with various adhesive resin cement combinations. *J. Prosthet. Dent.* **2018**, *119*, 826–832. [CrossRef]
19. Magne, P.; Belser, U. *Bonded Porcelain Restorations in the Anterior Dentition: A Biomimetic Approach*; Quintessence: Chicago, IL, USA, 2002.
20. Da Costa, D.C.; Coutinho, M.; de Sousa, A.S.; Ennes, J.P. A meta-analysis of the most indicated preparation design for porcelain laminate veneers. *J. Adhes. Dent.* **2013**, *15*, 215–220.
21. Abuzenada, B.; Alanazi, A.; Saydali, W.; Elmarakby, A.; Koshak, H.; Alharthi, A. Current classifications and preparation techniques of dental ceramic laminate veneers (Review article). *Int. J. Adv. Res.* **2017**, *5*, 1973–1979. [CrossRef]
22. Wells, D.J. "No-prep" veneers. *Inside Dent.* **2010**, *6*, 56–60.
23. Fradeani, M.; Redemagni, M.; Corrado, M. Porcelain laminate veneers: 6- to 12-year clinical evaluation-a retrospective study. *Int. J. Periodontics Restor. Dent.* **2005**, *25*, 9–17.

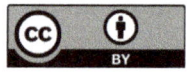

© 2019 by the authors. Licensee MDPI, Basel, Switzerland. This article is an open access article distributed under the terms and conditions of the Creative Commons Attribution (CC BY) license (http://creativecommons.org/licenses/by/4.0/).

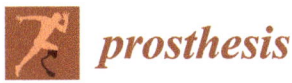

Article

An Integrated Approach, Orthodontic and Prosthetic, in a Case of Maxillary Lateral Incisors Agenesis

Marco Portelli *, Angela Militi, Antonino Logiudice and Riccardo Nucera

Department of Biomedical, Dental Science and Morphological and Functional Images, Dental School, University of Messina, Messina 98100, Italy; amiliti@unime.it (A.M.); nino.logiudice@gmail.com (A.L.); riccardon@unime.it (R.N.)
* Correspondence: mportelli@unime.it

Received: 28 July 2019; Accepted: 2 September 2019; Published: 4 September 2019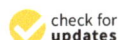

Abstract: Background: Among tooth anomalies, missing teeth is one of the most frequent, and it can be related to different therapeutical sets of problems. Often, an integrated approach that interests both orthodontists and prosthodontists is necessary, and in some cases also the periodontists. Methods: In this paper the authors report a clinical case of a 14-year-old patient, affected by maxillary bilateral incisors agenesis, molar bilateral II class and deep bite, treated in the Department of Orthodontics and Pedodontics of the University of Messina. The orthodontic treatment target was the distal movement of the maxillary molar, and the recovery of the space necessary for the prosthetic restoration of the missing lateral incisor. Maxillary molars distal movement was performed with a Distal Jet apparatus, skeletally supported by two miniscrews (Distal-Screw, American Orthodontics, Sheboygan, WI, USA). After molar relationship correction, a multi-bracket bimaxillary orthodontic appliance was bonded using Empower Brackets (American Orthodontics, Sheboygan, WI, USA). At the end of orthodontic treatment a Maryland bridge, bonded on the central incisors and cuspids, was used in order to maintain the space necessary for the insertion of dental implants in the region of 1.2 and 2.2. Results: A class II molar relationship was corrected, with an improvement of the deep bite, and the space necessary for implant insertion was recovered Conclusion: A skeletally supported Distal Jet was efficient for molar distalization, with the advantage of not having any loss of anchorage in the anterior part of the dental arch. This apparatus does not need patient compliance, have favorable aesthetics and also give the possibility to perform asymmetric activations.

Keywords: lateral incisors agenesis; space recovery; dental implants

1. Introduction

Tooth agenesis is probably the most frequent tooth anomaly and is strongly related to genetic patterns [1]. Maxillary lateral incisors agenesis incidence seems to be rather elevated, with values of about 6% [2]. Such a clinical condition is related to different therapeutic problems, and it is often necessary to have an integrated approach that interest both orthodontists and prosthodontists, and in some cases also the periodontists [3,4]. Teeth agenesis affects first of all the third molar, and then mandibular second premolar and maxillary lateral incisor, and among tooth agenesis the maxillary lateral incisor one is the more relevant, because of its significant impact on dental aesthetics. In cases of maxillary lateral incisors agenesis, a dental anomaly must be corrected as soon as possible, with space recovery if is it possible, in order to prevent functional effects. Differential diagnosis between impacted or a missing tooth can be obtained with a low dose CT acquisition, that provides more detailed diagnostic information without a significant increase in radiological risk for patients. If it is possible, orthodontic treatment targets the recovery of the anterior space, often lost because of the mesial shift of latero-posterior teeth; in such cases the first step of orthodontic treatment is molar distal movement. Several clinical conditions must be evaluated in order to decide if it is necessary to open or close the space for missing lateral maxillary incisors. A patient's facial aesthetics is one of the most important factors that must be considered, and if it is necessary to improve dental support to the upper lip, the recovery of the space is strongly recommended. In cases of a reduced vertical dimension, with dental deep-bite, the recovery of the space for missing lateral incisors, with molar distal movement, is recommended in order to produce a posterior rotation of the mandible and consequently an increase of the vertical dimension of the face and a correction of dental deep-bite. Maxillary molars distal movement can be obtained with both intra- and extraoral appliances. An intraoral apparatus offers the advantage of no patient compliance, however they could produce some side effects [5,6], especially in terms of anterior anchorage lost. A no compliance apparatus includes different types of devices, such as Distal jet, Pendulum, compressed coil springs, repelling magnets, etc. Intraoral devices can be skeletally supported in order to prevent loss of dental anchorage; this type of anchorage has been proposed for the first time by Creekmore in 1983 and Jenner in 1985, but nowadays several studies are available in the literature [7–9] about a skeletal-supported molar distalization apparatus. Dental anchorage represents the resistance to unwanted tooth movement, and can be classified in maximum, medium and minimum. Maximum anchorage corresponds to a complete absence of movement of the anchorage unit in consequence of reactive forces applied to other teeth [10]. Such anchorage can be obtained only if the anchorage apparatus is bone supported; an example is represented by miniplates, miniscrews, palatal implants and dental implants. There is no sufficient evidence in the literature about the efficiency and efficacy of different skeletal anchorage devices. For this reason, skeletal anchorage system selection is usually based on an individual preference of clinicians. In clinical practice miniscrews are the most commonly used because of their easily insertion and their elevated reported success rates, which is estimated around 80%–90% and similar to mini plate and palatal implant ones [11]. Different authors studied the ideal sites for miniscrew placement, and most of them proposed the palate as one of the better sites [12]. Palatal area offer both sufficient quality and quantity of bone for miniscrew insertion. However, the incisive canal region and the median area must be excluded, instead the para-median area present a cortical bone density and is thick enough to support the insertion of a miniscrew, and is able to bear orthopedic loads [13]. The para-median palatal area is devoid of sensible anatomical structures like blood vessels, nerves and dental root, which can create problems in miniscrew insertion. Moreover para-median palatal soft tissue thickness at the level of the third wrinkle is about 3.06 ± 0.45 mm^2: This thickness offers sufficient stability for miniscrew insertion. Para-median miniscrew insertion in growing children, moreover, does not interfere with growth processes at the level of the midpalatal suture [14].

2. Materials and Methods

We present a clinical case of a 14-year-old patient, male, with agenesis of the maxillary lateral incisors, a bilateral II class molar relationship and deep-bite. The patient turned to the Department of Orthodontics of Messina University for a dental visit, and an orthodontic check-up was performed with photographic reports (Figure 1), Panoramic Rx and L-L head teleradiography (Figure 2), as well as a cephalometric examination and comprehending also a facial aesthetic evaluation.

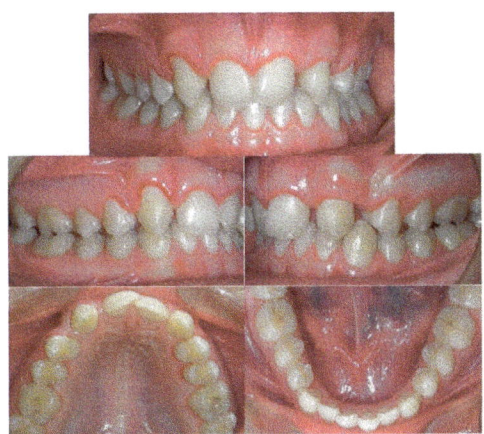

Figure 1. Pre-treatment intraoral reports.

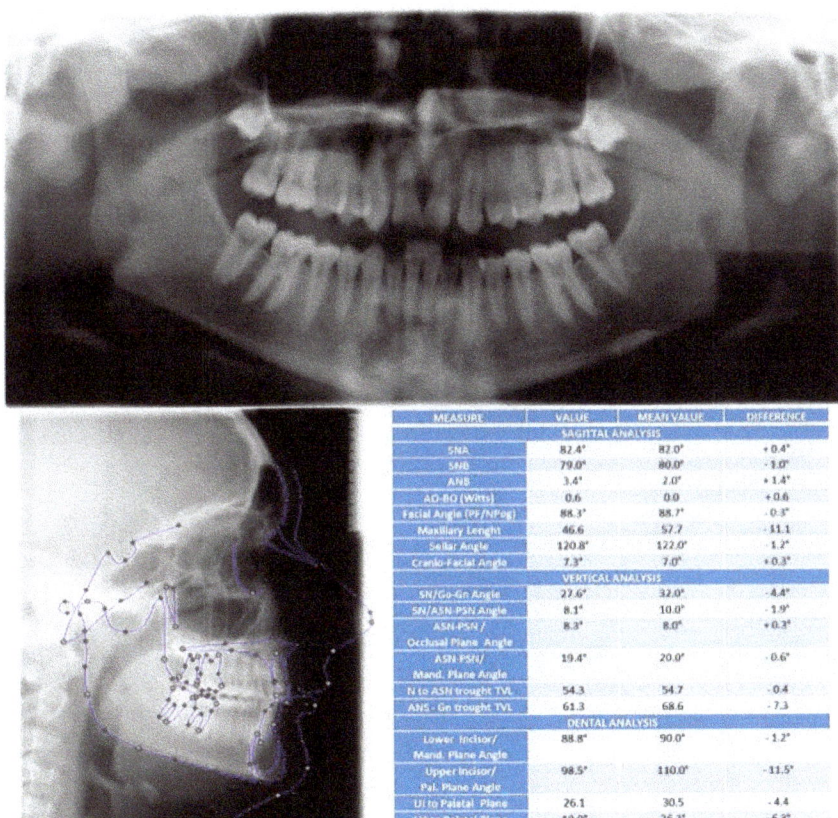

Figure 2. Pre-treatment X-ray exams.

Impressions in alginate of both arches was done and dental casts were obtained in order to perform dental discrepancies analysis [15]. In order to correct dental deep-bite and improve the patient's facial aesthetic, giving a better support to the upper lip, an orthodontic treatment plan predicted the recovery of the space necessary for the prosthetic restoration of lateral incisor agenesis. Maxillary molars distal movement as performed with a miniscrew skeletal-supported Distal Jet, called Distal-Screw (American Orthodontics, Sheboygan, WI, USA). The device presents two palatal coil springs whose compression generates forces with a distal vector over the first maxillary molars, and the effect of such forces produces distal movement of maxillary first molars. An accurate design of the apparatus and a favorable palatal anatomy, in this case produced a resultant line of forces close to the maxillary molar's center of resistance. A traditional Distal Jet produces a reactive force with undesired side effects on the anterior teeth. The use of a bone-anchored device eliminates the problems related to the reactive forces discharged on the anterior teeth, because they are absorbed by the maxillary bone [16]. The Distal-Screw was placed using two screws with an 11 mm length, inserted in the para-median area of the palate, and the maximum activation of the coil spring was done in order to perform maxillary molar distal movement and overcome the resistance offered by second and third maxillary molars (Figure 3).

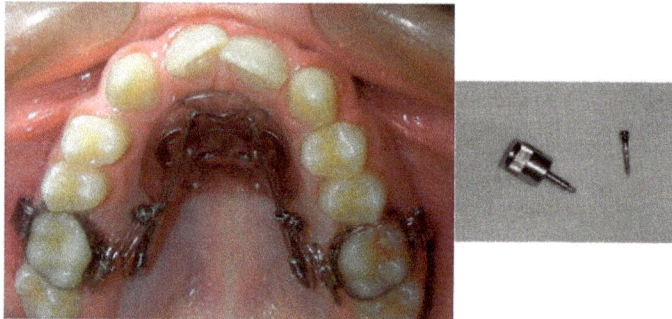

Figure 3. Palatal view of the Distal-Screw.

The miniscrew insertion procedure is really simple, as it does not need a gingival flap and can be performed with local anesthesia; in this case both the screws showed a good primary stability and was immediately loaded. The para-median palatal area is an ideal zone for TADS insertion, thanks to its easy access, the presence of keratinized soft tissues and a low risk of dental damage or vessels/nerve injury. Miniscrews must be inserted at the level of the third palatal wrinkle; several studies [17–19] report that this area can be considered as a safety zone for TADS insertion. Maxillary molar distal movement was completed in about seven months, reaching a bilateral molar I class relationship (Figure 4).

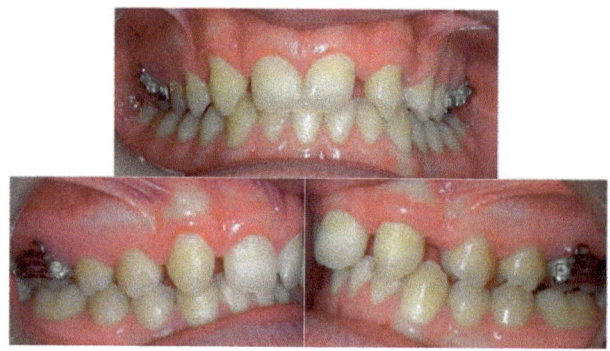

Figure 4. Molar relationship after Distal-Screw.

In order to lead the correction of maxillary molar distal tipping, with a greater distal movement of the crown compared to the root one, an overcorrection of the molar class relationship was done.

An orthodontic multi-bracket appliance was bonded and, in order to reduce the frictional forces between the slot and the arches and obtain a shorter treatment time [20,21], self-ligating mechanics were used (Empower, AO, Sheboygan, WI, USA) (Figure 5).

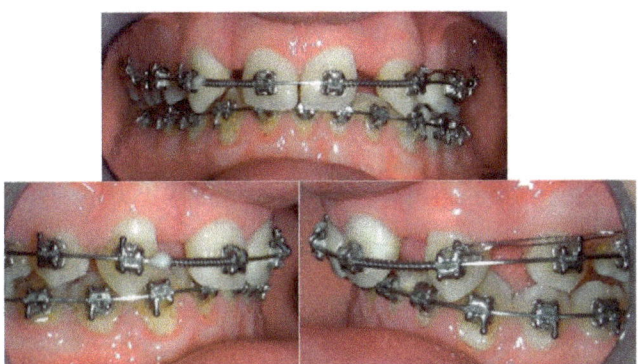

Figure 5. Self-ligating orthodontic appliance.

Once the initial phases of alignment and leveling were completed, an 0.017 inch × 0.025 inch Thermal Nickel–Titanium wire (American Orthodontics, Sheboygan, WI, USA) and two coil springs were positioned between the maxillary central incisors and cuspids, in order to produce canines' distal movement and complete the recovery of the space necessary for the prosthetic restoration of the lateral incisors agenesis. Once the canine distal movement was completed, with the achievement of a bilateral canine I class relationship, a traditional archwire sequence was done, with rectangular stainless-steel wires for a full Tip and Torque expression, and B-Titanium wires for occlusal finishing. After the debonding of the multibrackets appliance, a metallic fixed retainer canine-to-canine was bonded in the lower arch, instead of in the maxillary arch, in order to maintain the space recovered for the following insertion of the dental implant, and a Maryland bridge was bonded at the level of the lateral incisors (Figure 6).

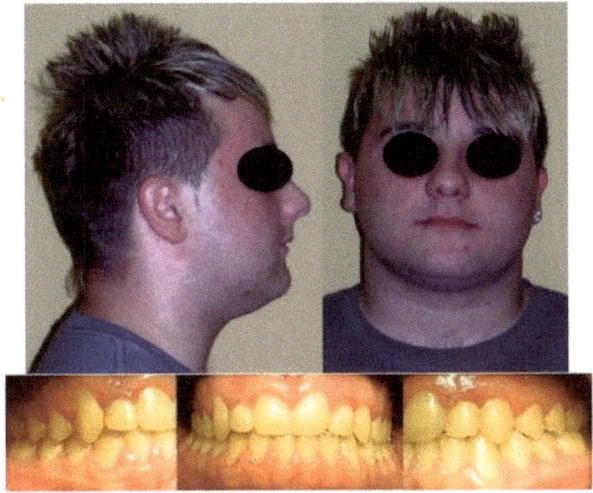

Figure 6. Post treatment.

3. Results

Thanks to the combined use of a skeletal-supported molar distalization apparatus and a multibracket self-ligating orthodontic appliance, in eighteen months of treatment the following clinical results were achieved: A bi-maxillary dental crowding correction, bilateral molars and cuspids I class relationship, overjet and overbite correction, dental midlines coincidence, occlusal plane correction, and recovery of the space necessary for the prosthetic restoration of maxillary lateral incisors agenesis.

4. Discussion

In the reported clinical case we decided to open the space necessary for the prosthetic restoration of lateral incisors agenesis in order to satisfy parents' request and above all for the correction of dental deep-bite and to improve the patient's facial aesthetic, giving a better support to the upper lip. The distal movement of maxillary molars provided a distal rotation of the mandible, with an increase in the facial vertical dimension and a correction of dental deep-bite. The effect of the no-compliance molar distalization device is a combination of distal crown movement and following tipping correction. Several factors can influence treatment results: Age, molar relationship (cusp–cusp or full II class) and the eruption of a second maxillary molar. Different studies support the hypothesis that molar distalization with a no-compliance apparatus is more efficient in cases of unerupted second molars. However, first molar distal movement is achievable also in cases where second molars have erupted [22]. In such cases, third molar extraction can be suggested. In the therapy note proposed in this study, first molar distal movement was reached, despite the age of the patient and the eruption of the second molars. A systematic review performed in 2011 by Fudalej and Antoszewska [23] regarding the effectiveness of an orthodontic distalizer reinforced with a temporary skeletal anchorage, demonstrated that a skeletally supported device reduces the side effect characteristics of a dental supported apparatus. This review moreover demonstrated that skeletal anchorage, both with implants, screws or miniplates, also increase the molar distalization rate, where Maxillary molars distal movement was between 3.9 mm and 6.4 mm without any loss of anchorage in the anterior part of the maxillary arch. Antonarikis and Kiliaridis [6] found in their systematic review that tooth-supported devices could produce a maxillary molar distal movement of about 2.9 mm with an undesired maxillary incisor mesial tipping of 1.8 mm. The amount of maxillary molar distal movement can be lost both for the necessary correction of crown distal tipping and a root mesial one, and during the following retraction of the anterior teeth. Skeletally anchored devices, differently than tooth-borne ones, can be used as a reinforcement for maxillary molar anchorage during the phase of anterior teeth retraction. A non-integrated temporary anchored device has to be preferred with respect to the osseo-integrated ones; the first one present several clinical advantages, such as simple insertion, immediate loading, a lower cost and less discomfort to the patients. A skeletal-supported device also reduces the possibility of side effects on the TMJ [24,25] characteristic of other devices with extra-dental discharge of reactive forces such as TEO. The pain induced by miniscrew insertion can be easily controlled with a common anti-inflammatory drug [26]. The disadvantages in the use of TAD can be represented by the necessity of a more detailed radiological investigation of the patient [27] and the risk for dental root and periapical damages [28].

5. Conclusions

According to the clinical outcomes obtained in the study case, the following conclusions can be affirmed:

- A skeletally anchored Distal Jet is effective and efficient for maxillary molar distal movement, offering the advantage of no side effects in the anterior part of the arch.
- The miniscrew insertion and removal procedure is really simple, fast and painless for the patient. Moreover, soft tissues have not developed inflammation or bleeding.
- Molar distal movement was obtained in a few months with a final distal tipping and rotation of the crowns; no vertical changes were observed.

- A distal screw presents several clinical advantages such as no patient compliance, good aesthetics, predictable outcomes and the possibility of asymmetric effects.
- Thanks to a specific design, a distal screw also allows the spontaneous distal drift of premolars induced by o transept periodontal fibers stretching.
- A distal screw can also be used as an anchorage device during the following phase of treatment of anterior teeth retraction, in order to avoid side effects on the maxillary molars.

Author Contributions: Conceptualization, M.P. and R.N.; methodology, A.L.; validation, A.L; formal analysis, A.M.; investigation, A.M.; data curation, A.L.; writing—original draft preparation, M.P.; writing—review and editing, M.P.; visualization, M.P.; supervision, R.N.

Funding: This research received no external funding.

Conflicts of Interest: The authors declare no conflict of interest

References

1. Militi, D.; Militi, A.; Cutrupi, M.C.; Portelli, M.; Rigoli, L.; Matarese, G.; Salpietro, D.C. Genetic basis of non syndromic hypodontia: A DNA investigation performed on three couples of monozygotic twins about PAX9 mutation. *Eur. J. Paed Dent.* **2011**, *12*, 21–24.
2. Militi, A.; Vitale, C.; Portelli, M.; Matarese, G.; Cordasco, G. Open bite anteriore con agenesia dei secondi premolari inferiori: Terapia estrattiva con utilizzo di attacchi auto leganti. *Mondo Ortod.* **2012**, *37*, 1–15. [CrossRef]
3. Worsaae, N.; Jensen, B.N.; Holm, B.; Holsko, J. Tretament of severe hypodontia-oligodontia an interdisciplinary concept. *Int. J. Oral Maxillofac. Surg.* **2007**, *36*, 266–269. [CrossRef] [PubMed]
4. Vitale, C.; Militi, A.; Portelli, M.; Cordasco, G.; Matarese, G. Maxillary Canine-First Premolar transposition in the permanent dentition. *J. Clin. Orth.* **2009**, *8*, 517–523.
5. Chiu, P.P.; McNamara, J.A., Jr.; Franchi, L. A comparison of two intraoral molar distalization appliances: Distal jet versus pendulum. *Am. J. Orthod. Dentofac. Orthop.* **2005**, *128*, 353–365. [CrossRef]
6. Antonarakis, G.S.; Kiliaridis, S. Maxillary molar distalization with non compliance intramaxillary appliances in Class II malocclusion. A systematic review. *Angle Orthod.* **2008**, *78*, 1133–1140. [CrossRef] [PubMed]
7. Gelgor, I.E.; Buyukyilmaz, T.; Karaman, A.I.; Dolanmaz, D.; Kalayci, A. Intraosseus screw-supported upper molar distalization. *Angle Orthod.* **2004**, *74*, 838–850. [PubMed]
8. Kinzinger, G.S.; Gulden, N.; Yildizhan, F.; Diedrich, P.R. Efficiency of a skeletonized distal jet appliance supported by miniscrew anchorage for non compliance maxillary molar distalization. *Am. J. Orthod. Dentofac. Orthop.* **2009**, *136*, 578–586. [CrossRef]
9. Papadopoulos, M.A.; Melkos, A.B.; Athanasiou, A.E. Non compliance maxillary molar distalization with the first class appliance: A randomized controlled trial. *Am. J. Orthod. Dentofac. Orthop.* **2010**, *137*, 586–587. [CrossRef]
10. Daskalogiannakis, J. *Glossary of Orthodontic Terms Leipzig*; Quintessence Publishing Co.: Batavila, IL, USA, 2000.
11. Tsui, W.K.; Chua, H.D.P.; Cheung, L.K. Bone anchor systems for orthodontic application: A systematic review. *Int. J. Oral Maxillofac. Surg.* **2012**, *41*, 1427–1438. [CrossRef]
12. Poggio, P.M.; Incorvati, C.; Velo, S.; Carano, A. Safe zones: A guide for miniscrew positioning in the maxillary and mandibular arch. *Angle Orthod.* **2006**, *76*, 191–197. [PubMed]
13. Martina, R.; Cioffi, I.; Farella, M.; Leone, P.; Manzo, P.; Matarese, G.; Portelli, M.; Nucera, R.; Cordasco, G. Transverse changes determined by rapid and slow maxillary expansion—A low-dose CT-based randomized controlled trial. *Orthod. Cranio Facial. Res.* **2012**, *15*, 159–168. [CrossRef] [PubMed]
14. Schauseil, M.; Ludwig, B.; Zorkun, B.; Hellak, A.; Korbmacher-Steiner, H. Density of the midpalatal suture after RME treatment—A retrospective comparative low-dose CT-study. *Head Face Med.* **2014**, *10*, 18. [CrossRef] [PubMed]
15. Portelli, M.; Matarese, G.; Militi, A.; Cordasco, G.; Lucchese, A. A proportional correlation index for space analysis in mixed dentition derived from an Italian population sample. *Eur. J. Paed Dent.* **2012**, *13*, 113–117.
16. Kinzinger, G.S.M.; Diedrich, P.R.; Bowman, S.J. Upper molar distalization with a miniscrew-supported distal jet. *J. Clin. Orthod.* **2006**, *40*, 672–678. [PubMed]

17. Seong, H.; Bayome, M.; Lee, J.; Lee, J.Y.; Song, H.H.; Kook, Y.A. Evaluation of palatal bone density in adults and adolescent for application of skeletal anchorage devices. *Angle Orthod.* **2012**, *4*, 625–631.
18. Matarese, G.; Portelli, M.; Mazza, M.; Militi, A.; Nucera, R.; Gatto, E.; Cordasco, G. Evaluation of skin dose in a low dose spiral CT protocol. *Eur. J. Paed Dent.* **2006**, *7*, 77–80.
19. Cordasco, G.; Portelli, M.; Militi, A.; Nucera, R.; Lo Giudice, A.; Gatto, E.; Lucchese, A. Low-dose protocol of the spiral CT in orthodontics: Comparative evaluation of entrance skin dose with traditional X-ray techniques. *Prog. Orthod.* **2013**, *10*, 14–24.
20. Lucchese, A.; Bertacci, A.; Chersoni, S.; Portelli, M. Primary enamel permeability:a SEM evaluation in vivo. *Eur. J. Ped Dent.* **2012**, *13*, 231–235.
21. Matarese, G.; Nucera, R.; Militi, A.; Mazza, M.; Portelli, M.; Festa, F.; Cordasco, G. Evaluation of frictional forces during dental alignment: An experimental model with 3 nonleveled brackets. *Am. J. Orthod. Dentofac. Orthop.* **2008**, *133*, 708–715. [CrossRef]
22. Kinzinger, G.S.; Fritz, U.B.; Sander, F.G.; Diedrich, P.R. Efficiency of a pendulum appliance for molar distalization related to second and thrird molar eruption stage. *Am. J. Orthod. Dentofac. Orthop.* **2004**, *125*, 8–23. [CrossRef] [PubMed]
23. Fudalej, P.; Antoszewska, J. Are orthodontic distalizers reinforced with temporary skeletal anchorage devices effective? *Am. J. Orthod. Dentofac. Orthop.* **2011**, *139*, 722–729. [CrossRef] [PubMed]
24. Portelli, M.; Matarese, G.; Militi, A.; Logiudice, G.; Nucera, R.; Lucchese, A. Temporomandibular joint involvement in a cohort of patients with juvenile idiopathic arthritis and evaluation of the effect induced by functional orthodontic appliance: Clinical and radiographic investigation. *Eur. J. Paed Dent.* **2014**, *15*, 63–66.
25. Portelli, M.; Gatto, E.; Matarese, G.; Militi, A.; Catalfamo, L.; Gherlone, E.; Lucchese, A. Unilateral condylar hyperplasia: Diagnosis, clinical aspects and operative treatment. A case report. *Eur. J. Paed Dent.* **2015**, *16*, 99–102.
26. Scolari, G.; Lazzarin, F.; Fornaseri, C.; Rengo, S.; Amato, M.; Cicciù, D.; Braione, D.; Morgantini, A.; Bassetti, C.; Tramér, M.; et al. A comparison of Nimesulide Beta Cyclodextrin and Nimesulide in postoperative dental pain. *Int. J. Clin. Pract.* **1999**, *53*, 345–348. [PubMed]
27. Di Lorenzo, P.; Niola, M.; Pantaleo, G.; Buccelli, C.; Amato, M. On the comparison of age determination methods based on dental development radiographic studies in a sample of Italian population. *Dental Cadmos* **2015**, *83*, 38–45. [CrossRef]
28. Paduano, S.; Uomo, R.; Amato, M.; Riccitiello, F.; Simeone, M.; Valletta, R. Cyst-like periapical lesion healing in an orthodontic patient: A case report with five-year follow-up. *G. Ital. Endod.* **2013**, *27*, 95–104. [CrossRef]

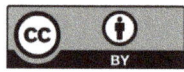

© 2019 by the authors. Licensee MDPI, Basel, Switzerland. This article is an open access article distributed under the terms and conditions of the Creative Commons Attribution (CC BY) license (http://creativecommons.org/licenses/by/4.0/).

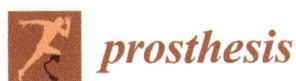

Case Report

Implant-Supported Prosthetic Therapy of an Edentulous Patient: Clinical and Technical Aspects

Luca Ortensi [1],*, Marco Ortensi [2], Andrea Minghelli [3] and Francesco Grande [4]

1 Department of Prosthodontics, University of Catania, 95124 Catania, Italy
2 CDT Private Practice, 40126 Bologna, Italy; centro.odontotecnico@tiscali.it
3 School of Dentistry, University of Bologna, 40126 Bologna, Italy; andrea.minghelli2@studio.unibo.it
4 Oral and Maxillofacial Surgery, University of Bologna, 40126 Bologna, Italy; francesco.grande6@unibo.it
* Correspondence: luca.ortensi@unict.it

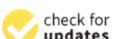

Received: 20 May 2020; Accepted: 23 June 2020; Published: 1 July 2020

Abstract: The purpose of this article is to show how to implement an implant-supported prosthetic overdenture using a digital workflow. Esthetic previewing using a specific software, guided-surgery, construction of the prosthesis, and the esthetic finalization are described in this article. Patients suffering from severe loss of bone and soft tissue volume could benefit from the construction of an overdenture prosthesis as a feasible therapeutic choice for functional and esthetic issues of the patient.

Keywords: prosthesis; Digital Smile System; overdenture; digital prosthetic planning; atrophic patient

1. Introduction

A pleasant appearance is ever more aspired to in the daily life of everyone, at any age. When adverse changes occur to a visible part of the body, the social and psychological impact can be negative for the individual [1]. Among the least well-tolerated changes is edentulism; which, in addition to causing significant functional deficits (chewing, phonetics), involves visible changes of facial esthetics, because with the loss of teeth and the resulting reabsorption of the alveolar crests, there is naturally less support for the soft tissues of the face, which takes on an unpleasant look, regardless of the person's age. Although the total removable prosthetic is doable in a short timeframe and is economical and efficient, it is not easy to make to enhance the function and esthetics of the totally edentulous patient. These two aspects are certainly an advantage, but that is not enough to consider removable prosthesis for the ideal prosthetic therapy. In fact, not even this type of state-of-the-art prosthetic can completely restore chewing capacity and strength in some types of patients [2]. In elderly patients with atrophic maxilla, the implant-supported removable prosthesis (overdenture) is considered a feasible option in the prosthetic treatment plan [3]. When a severe loss of supporting bone structure has already happened, it would be necessary to optimize the soft tissues aspect of the lower third of the face, facilitating, at the same time, home oral hygiene procedures and patient comfort [4,5]. Stabilization of the removable prosthesis with a reduced number of implants may present multiple advantages. The biological and economic costs could be contained, the time for oral rehabilitation is shorter, and the long-term success rates are over 90%. In the mandible, two implants seem to be sufficient to obtain good stabilization of the removable prosthesis and the literature does not show statistically significant differences in terms of survival rate and comfort for the patient between insertion of two or four implants, solidified by a bar or with connections not constraining the implants (i.e., ball-attachment or other individual attachment type) [6]. On the other hand, for the upper maxilla the insertion of only two implants is not considered an ideal option if long cantilevers are expected; more predictable results could be achieved with the insertion of at least four implants connected by a metal or titanium bar, considering also the shape of the maxillary arch [7]. In this specific therapy, the prosthesis could have a limited palate, improving the patient's comfort and flavor perception [8].

However, the treatment plan of atrophic patients is a challenging procedure for the clinician and also the technician. Several factors should be considered during the treatment planning in order to realize an appropriate oral rehabilitation.

Recently modern prosthetics makes use of digital technologies to support both the diagnostic and the therapeutic phases of patient rehabilitation, facilitating also the communication between the clinician and the lab [9–11].

Traditional removable prosthetics and those supported by implants have benefitted from these innovations both in virtual planning of clinical cases and as a support during the construction phase [12–15].

The purpose of this article is to illustrate, through detailed step-by-step description of a complex clinical case, the construction of an inferior overdenture with implant support, applying the new digital technologies to every phase of the diagnostic and prosthetic therapy, reducing implementation time and analogical phases.

2. Materials and Methods

A 70-year old patient came to the dental office complaining of diminished masticatory capacity and loss of retention of both removable dentures. She wanted to improve her smile and facial esthetics, stating she was dissatisfied with the color and poor visibility of her teeth, no matter how big she smiled. The patient also asked to avoid multiple-steps therapies and desired to have a new prosthetic solution in the shortest time as possible. The patient's smile seemed non-harmonious due to dental wear and the inclination of the occlusal planes, which affected her general appearance (Figure 1). The patient gave her written consent to publish photos of her clinical case, including photos of her face.

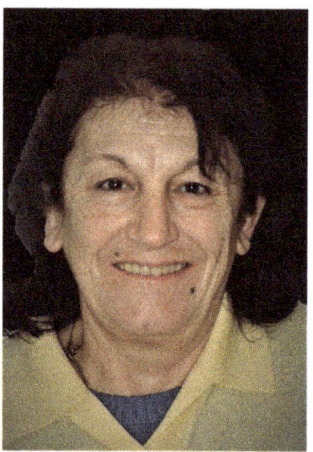

Figure 1. Initial state of the face: a reduction of the vertical dimension is observed with an increase in perilabial wrinkles.

Her history did not show any pathology incompatible with dental treatment and demonstrated that she was in good general health and classified as ASA1. The facial examination showed a reduction of the vertical dimension, with a widening of the nasolabial folds, and diminished tone of the perioral soft tissue, with a generalized deterioration of all facial esthetic parameters (Figure 2). During the intraoral clinical examination, incongruous prosthesis in both arches have been observed (Figure 3).

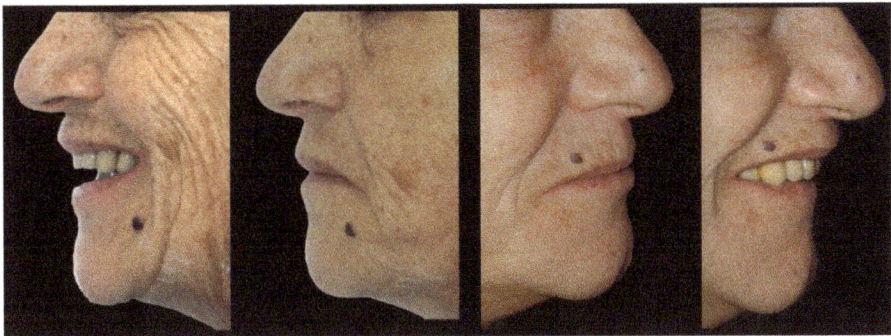

Figure 2. Extraoral facial photos: lateral view.

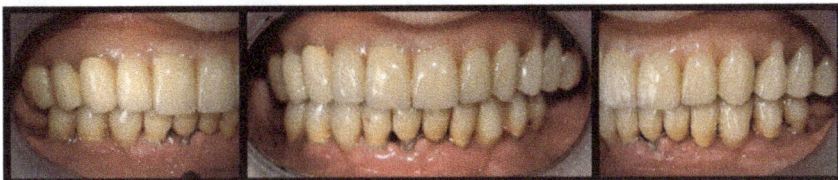

Figure 3. Intraoral photos of the removable dentures.

The upper arch had a full-removable denture, while the lower jaw had a fixed prosthesis supported by few periodontally compromised teeth as shown by the periapical mandibular radiographs, which also show several periodontal pockets, different carious lesions, and bone resorption around the natural abutments (Figure 4).

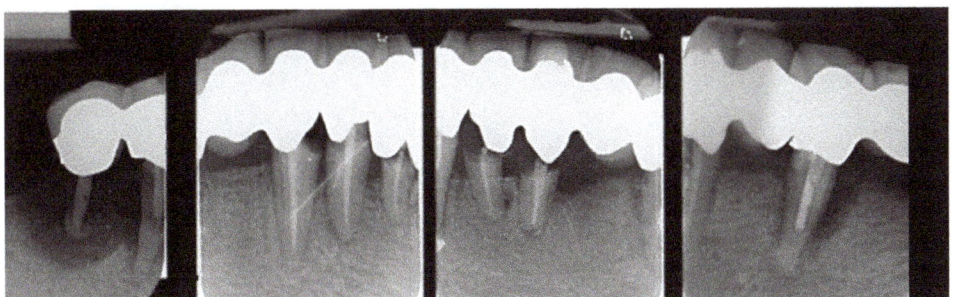

Figure 4. Endoral periapical radiographs of mandibular teeth.

During the first visit, several instrumental analyses were done, such as lateral cephalometric and electromyography. Lateral cephalometry is a valuable diagnostic tool that the authors consider pivotal for formulating a proper treatment plan in a complex prosthetic rehabilitation of an atrophic patient [16]. This x-ray examination enables the study of the hard and soft tissues of the patient's face; in particular, the relationship between the maxilla as well as the spatial position of the upper central incisor and the philtrum. It is also possible to identify the musculoskeletal classification with an appropriate and simple cephalometric analysis [17]. The study of the patient's latero–lateral radiography highlighted meso-facial musculoskeletal typology with reduced occlusal risk. Surface electromyography, using electrodes placed on the masticatory muscles, will allow the clinician to evaluate masticatory activity and to understand whether the occlusal load is adequate or excessive [18]. A measurement of chewing loads produced by the patient is not a secondary element; on the contrary it represents an important aspect of comparison for the whole working group, and in particular with the dental technician who will have to take into consideration the extent of these values during the design and construction of the prosthesis.

In the first appointment two photos were taken of the patient's face according to a coded technique for the DSS (Digital Smile System, Bologna, Italy) software [19]. It is important to take photos of the face keeping the patient in a position that is stable and repeatable over time, trying not to change the enlargement ratio between shots. For this purpose, the patient is asked to sit comfortably keeping her back straight while the operator used a camera set on a tripod to stabilize its position in relation to the patient being photographed. The subject had to be positioned so that their Frankfurt Plane (the line that joins the Porion and the Orbital Point) was parallel to the horizon. Once the spatial position of the head is identified, it must remain unchanged with respect to the camera-tripod complex. The patient may wear dedicated glasses used to calibrate the digital pre-rendering software (DSS; Figure 5).

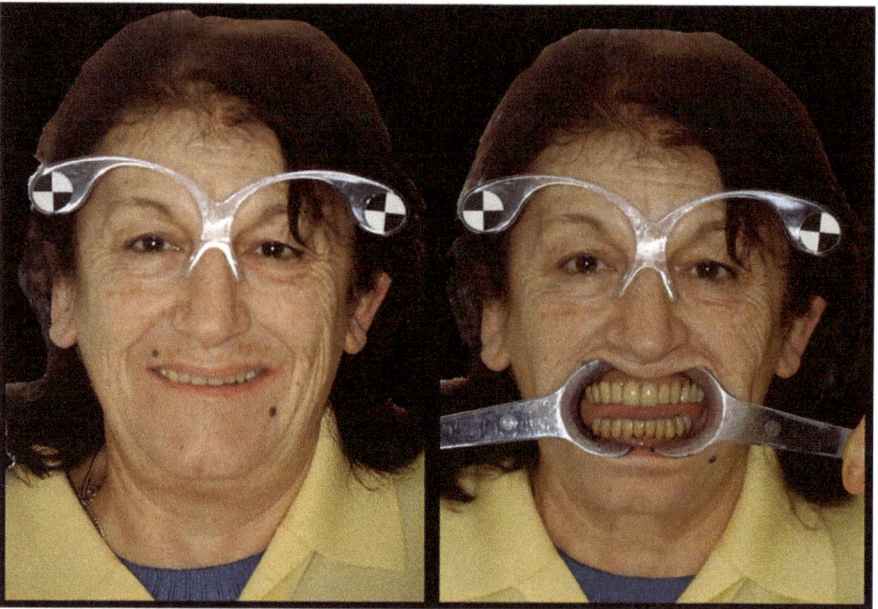

Figure 5. The first facial photo was taken asking the patient to smile and show as many teeth as possible and the second facial photograph was taken with cheek retractors.

The glasses represent a true measuring system that differentiates this software from other similar systems. Thanks to their shape and the presence of calibration markers used as a reference, the glasses facilitate maintenance of the perpendicular position of the patient and the camera. The first facial photo was taken asking the patient to smile and show as much teeth as possible. The second facial photograph was taken with cheek retractors to better highlight the teeth of the patient.

The photographic status is completed with the profile shots of her face and with the intraoral photographs that allow us to make further diagnostic assessments regarding the overall esthetics of her face and its physiognomic characteristics on which we can proceed with our prosthetic therapy [20]. After this phase, the two extraoral photos taken during the first visit were inserted in a dedicated 2D software (Digital Smile System, Bologna, Italy) useful for the final esthetic of the patient.

The Digital Smile System approach using digital techniques for the esthetic preview was only considered a tool for communication with the patient and for the entire dental team. DSS not only allowed the patient to see the esthetic future appearance, but it also enabled production of a prototype for the functional check of the digital project carried out [21]. The fact that the patient can see the possible future esthetic results through digital rendering, including the possibility of changes if desired, reduces overall clinical practice time. The procedure requires that the photographs taken be imported into the DSS and then an esthetic preview of the future prosthetic therapy is developed (Figure 6), which consists of a virtual arrangement of commercial teeth present in the software database. The database consists of upper and lower teeth of various shapes and sizes. Anterior and posterior teeth are positioned using the occlusal rim, previously suitably adapted in the oral cavity as a guide. Teeth are chosen according to esthetic and functional parameters and can be replaced with others of different shape or color, if necessary. This allows us to show the patient the possible final esthetic so that she can participate in the therapeutic project in collaboration with the whole clinical–technical team.

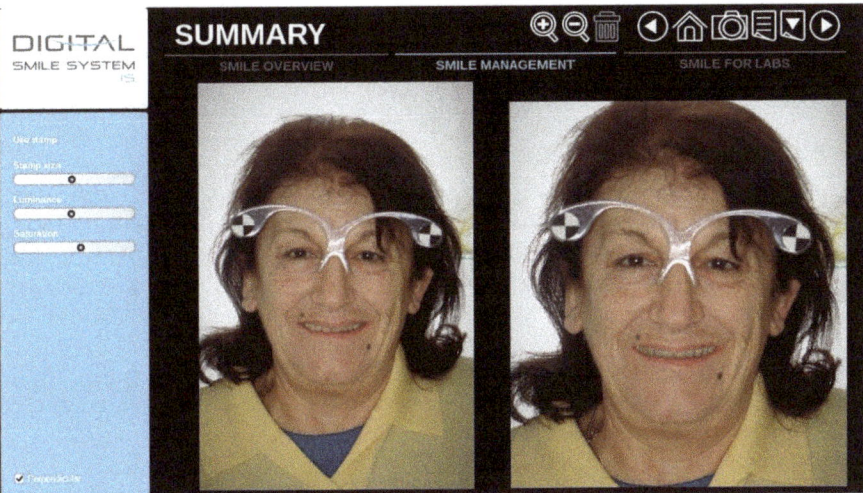

Figure 6. Digital preview of the final esthetic in the DSS software (2D).

In a dedicated appointment, all the compromised dental elements in the lower arch were extracted except the lateral incisor which serves as a provisional anchor of the new provisional lower denture (Figure 7).

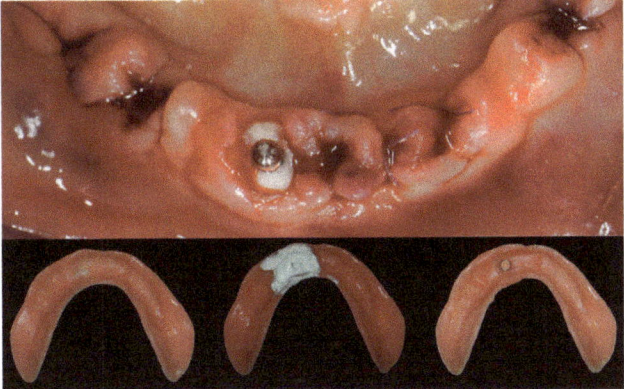

Figure 7. Use of lateral incisor as a provisional anchor for the provisional denture.

After tissue healing, preliminary impressions of the soft tissue and edentulous arches were made. The authors did not use an intraoral scanner (IOS) because there is no consensus in the literature regarding real efficacy in edentulous subjects [22]. We usually use a high-precision alginate with long setting time useful for tissue functionalization applied in two stages, where possible (only in edentulous subjects): a first impression is made with the alginate mixed with a high consistency (Neocolloid, Zhermack, Badia Polesine, Ro, Italy), it is then dried and modified by removing the undercut parts with a sharp tool and relined with the same material but in a more fluid form to read all the details of the anatomical tissues. The model obtained is scanned with a laboratory scanner (Sinergia Scan, Nobil Metal, Asti, Italy) and a resin occlusion base is built on it by sending a dedicated file to the 3D printer (Asiga MaxUV, Australia), coating it with wax for registration of the centric relationship, esthetic, functional determinants, and vertical dimension [23].

It is important in the upper occlusal rim, during functionalization in the oral cavity, to mark some landmarks; the midline, the canine line, and the smile line. These reference lines will serve in the alignment phase of the occlusal rims in the 3D software (Exocad software, Exocad GmbH, Darmstadt, Germany).

Transfer of Data from the Dental Office to the Laboratory

Once the virtual teeth arrangement was obtained—and approved by the patient—the file containing the patient's information, the photographic alignments, the libraries chosen, and the work process was transferred to the dental technician laboratory where the file was imported into a 3D software program (Exocad® software, Exocad GmbH). The information file exported from DSS consisted of a PDF format and individual photographs of the patient's face with a customized two-dimensional (2D) virtual smile design.

The files from DSS were then superimposed onto scanned images of the denture. The dental technician used the outline of the virtual smile obtained to place a tooth from the library or to create customized teeth with tools from Freeform (Exocad® software, Exocad GmbH) to convert the virtual 2D teeth arrangement into a 3D teeth arrangement [24].

Simply put, "coupling" of the data, thinking that the final image of the mounting, obtained in the 2D version, represents a face of the volumetric solid corresponding to what is in the 3D version (Figure 8).

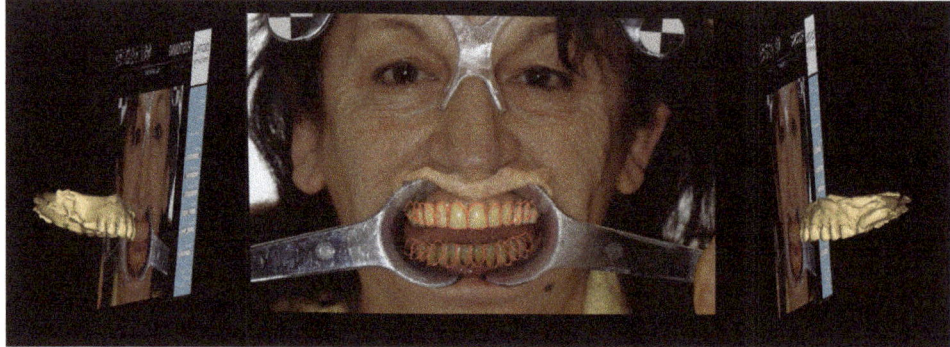

Figure 8. Overlap of the 2D image of the patient's face with the 3D digital model inside a 3D software. The 2D teeth represent the anterior face of the 3D solid.

The teeth used from the 3D database represent the volume of the solid, and the 2D teeth are the anterior face of this solid. The dental technician completes the 3D phase, improving the occlusal ratio between the arches (according to the literature) and producing the prosthetic base that will sustain the dental elements. After this phase, CAD (Computer-Aided Design) work can produce a prototype that corresponds entirely to the project made with DSS and processed in a 3D environment. The file obtained is sent to a 3D printer (Asiga MaxUV, Australia) and transformed into a prototype to be tested in the oral cavity, verifying the intraoral adaptation, the cranio–mandibular ratio, the esthetics of the smile and face. These prototypes represent the final volume of the final prosthesis. The clinician can make changes without impacting the protocol, in the prototypes, thus modified, can be scanned again by the technician, and overlapped digitally to the original project.

Subsequently the prototype is used as a radiological stent with which the CBCT(cone beam computed tomography) is done, using a dedicated device (Evobite with 3D marker, 3Diemme, Italy), which was adapted to the item with radiotransparent silicon (Elite Glass, Zhermack, Badia Polesine, Ro, Italy; Figure 9).

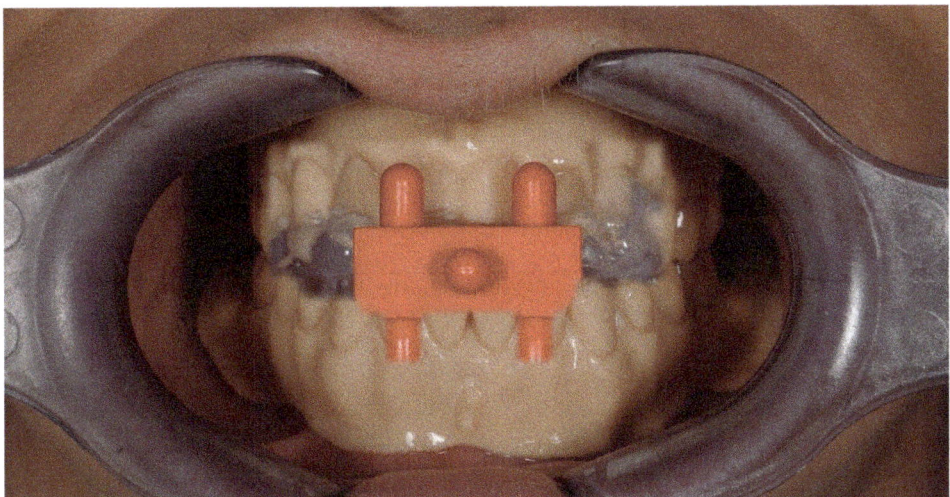

Figure 9. The prototype used as a radiological stent during the conduct of the CBCT (cone beam computed tomography).

The Dicom data resulting from the X-ray and the STL (Standard Triangulation Language) files relative to the anatomical and prosthetic parts obtained from the intraoral scan are imported in a specific implant planning software (Realguide 5.0, 3Diemme, Italy) where, thanks to a dedicated algorithm, they are overlapped using a replicable and controlled procedure. Through use of the implant line database (Thommen Medical AG, Grenchen, Switzerland), the number and position of the implant screws to be inserted via guided surgery are planned. After careful functional and esthetic evaluation and final verification, the prosthetic-driven plan was approved, and a stereolithographic surgical template was made using a newer rapid prototyping technology (New Ancorvis, Bargellino, Italy). Subsequently two prosthetic-driven implants with a diameter of 4.0 mm and a length of 9.5 mm (SPI ® CONTACT RC INICELL®, Thommen Medical AG) were placed, with a dedicated burr kit (Thommen Medical Guided Surgery Kit), in the lower jaw, taking into account the bone quality and quantity, soft-tissue thickness, anatomical landmarks, and the type, volume, and shape of the final restoration. The lateral incisor that acts as provisional anchor for the lower denture, in this phase was maintained in the mouth of the patient for the time necessary for implant loading. Healing screws are positioned directly post-surgically, and the prosthesis is readapted with resilient material (Coe-Soft™ GC America Inc., Alsip, IL, USA).

About four weeks later [25], after tissue healing, with a dedicated tool (Cuff Height Measuring Tool, Rhein 83, Bologna, Italy), measurements of the transmucosal paths were performed and the most suitable retention systems means were chosen (OT Equator, Rhein 83, Bologna, Italy; Figure 10) and were screwed to the implant fixtures with a preset force, with the corresponding retentive copings. The provisional prosthesis is readapted to make it suitable to receive the stainless-steel retentive cap housing nylon retentive inserts, improving the stability and hold. The general rule to apply for the choice of this type of attachments is the retentive part, which must extend beyond the transmucosal path by at least one millimeter [26].

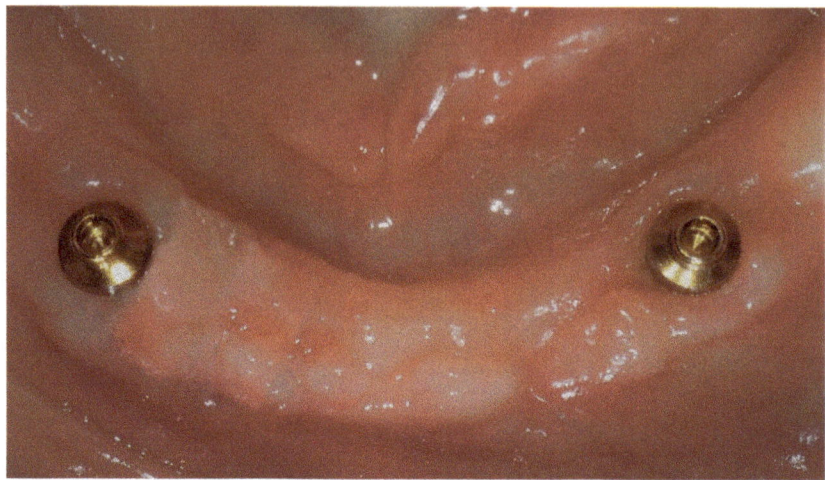

Figure 10. Equator attachments used to improve the stability and retention of prosthesis.

Thereafter the dental technician, using a 3D software (Exocad®, Exocad GmbH), plans the counter-bar [27], inserting retentive pins into the project for the mechanical hold of the teeth and preparing the area of the OT Equator attachment components (Rhein 83, Bologna, Italy).

The project is sent to the milling center (New Ancorvis, Bologna, Italia) indicating the type of metal to be used and the type of construction (laser melting technology). After being checked in the dental laboratory and sent to dentist for clinical testing, the precision and passivity of the piece is checked. The commercial teeth are then mounted, taking advantage of the prototype as a positioning guide. The perfectly polished prostheses are sent to the dental office (Figures 11–13), making sure there are no compression areas on the soft tissues. The patient is provided guidelines for prosthesis hygiene maintenance procedures.

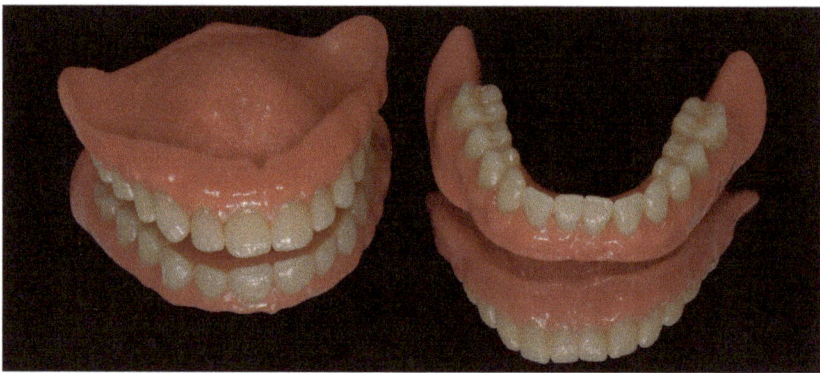

Figure 11. Details of the finished prosthesis.

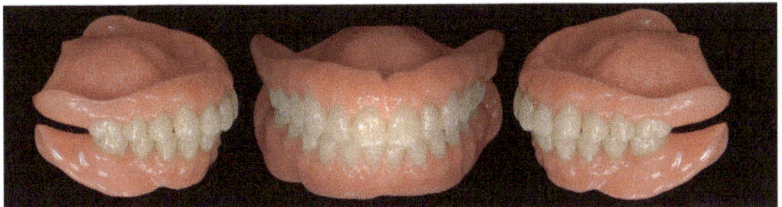

Figure 12. Completed dentures ready to be sent to the dental office.

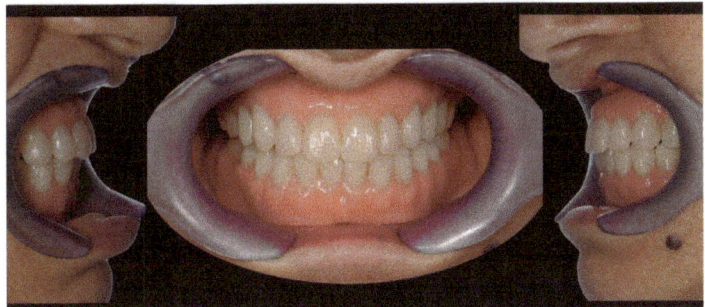

Figure 13. Postoperative intraoral view showing the good esthetic integration.

Once the prosthetic therapy was completed, the patient's face improved greatly from an esthetic viewpoint (Figure 14). The soft tissue of the face looked firm and toned. A reduction could be seen in the nasolabial folds and perilabial wrinkles (Figure 15), both frontally and laterally. The vertical dimension, which was slightly increased, appeared adequate and well-tolerated esthetically. During phonation and smiling dynamics the patient displayed natural looking teeth that were perfectly integrated with his face (Figure 16).

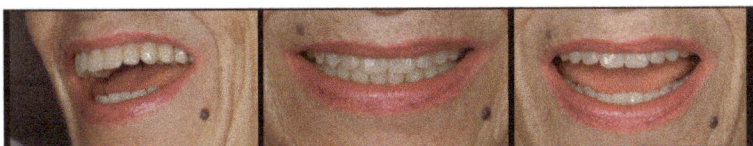

Figure 14. Patient's final smile with proper teeth position.

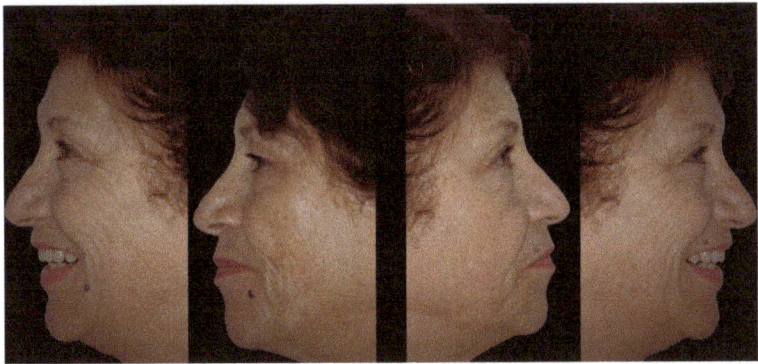

Figure 15. Patient's face in lateral view: the lip support appears correct.

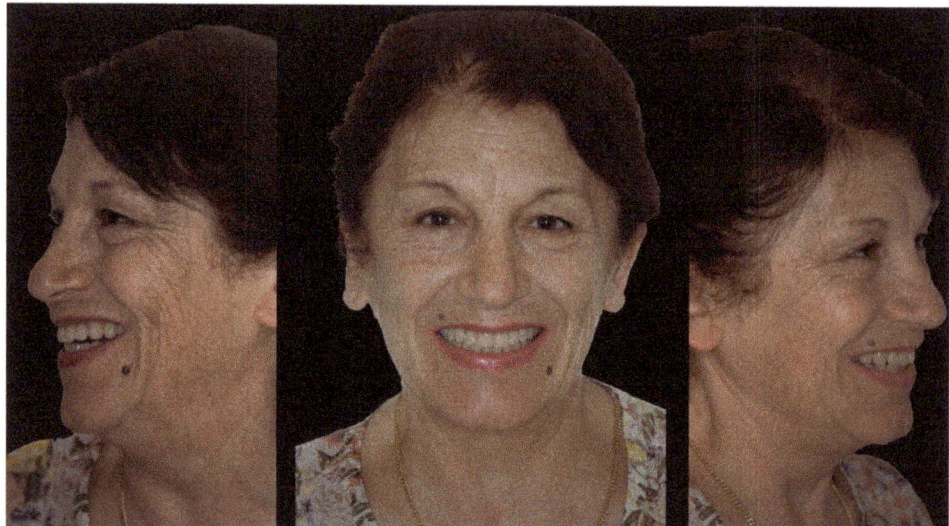

Figure 16. Patient's face at the end of the therapy: notice a reduction in the nasolabial folds and perilabial wrinkles.

3. Discussion

During the prosthetic therapy, for both fixed and removable prostheses, communication with the patient is a vital part of the treatment. Effective digital previewing is the ideal way to explain esthetic changes to a patient and to receive their approval. Until now, many digital previewing methods have been used in dentistry solely for this purpose. The authors deem that digital previewing of the smile must be inserted into a more complex workflow [28].

In this article, the Digital Smile System approach was introduced into a complex digital workflow. DSS (Digital Smile System, Bologna, Italy) not only allowed the patient to see their future appearance, but it also enabled production of a prototype for the functional check of the digital project carried out. The fact that the patient can see the possible future esthetic results through digital rendering, including the possibility of changes if desired, reduces overall clinical practice time. Additionally, the construction of a prototype, based on the virtual assembly, minimizes the number of errors in the manufacture of the final product and becomes a fundamental instrument for prosthetic-driven surgery. The decision-making process of using an implant overdenture prosthesis or a Toronto or hybrid prosthetic devices depends on different factors. The selection and extent of artificial tissues are related to facial support, emergence profile of the artificial tooth, the tooth angulation and the use of full flange extension is mentioned for esthetic advantages. However, the application of gingival prostheses may be limited to certain clinical situations where oral hygiene is manageable, function proper and esthetics acceptable. With a removable design, a larger volume of tissue can be replaced, and proper cleaning is still feasible. An instrument that could suggest a correct therapeutic choice is the latero–lateral radiography of the patient, which provides some important parameters: acrylic flange height, mucosal coverage, crown-Implant distance, and buccal prosthesis profile [16]. According to Avrampou et al., when the mucosal coverage is less than 5 mm and the prosthetic profile is up to 30 degrees, a fixed prosthesis whit hybrid or crown design can be selected. On the other hand, when the mucosal coverage is more than 5 mm and the prosthetic profile is less than 30 degrees, a removable prosthesis with a buccal flange is advised.

The use of overdenture involves different advantages. Compared to complete removable dentures, implant supported dentures have better stability and retention, improving function, esthetic, and satisfaction for the patient [29,30]. Furthermore, some data indicate that after receiving implants, patients with overdenture eat a diet with more fiber and hard foods than with conventional dentures, even if this does not improve nutritional intakes of essential micronutrients and macronutrients [31]. Furthermore, phonetic problems have been reported more often with fixed prostheses than with overdentures, probably because impaired phonetics appears to depend also on the palatal design of the prosthesis [32,33].

Use of the prototype as a radiological stent during the examination of the CBCT, and its transformation into a surgery-driven guide make it possible to position implants according to the digital study done with the DSS and approved by the patient. Some phases of the described workflow require a learning curve by the clinical operator and technician. For example, the photos taken by the clinician for the DSS, must be taken in the exact manner as previously described to facilitate superimposing of the photo of the patient's face, with the scan of the model and the old denture. Another important stage is ensuring the teeth from the database of the 3D software are matched with the outlines obtained by digital previewing with the DSS. In this case, if the match is not precise, the prototype will not correspond perfectly with that approved by the patient [34].

4. Conclusions

The use of digital technologies is now vastly widespread in the field of dentistry and, in particular, in prosthetic therapy. In removable, traditional, and implant-supported prosthetic therapy, digital technology can play an essential role. The clinical case described was almost entirely done with an innovative digital workflow, both from clinical and technical viewpoints. In particular, guided surgery came into the digital workflow through a simplified approach that was closely dependent on the patient's esthetics and functional aspects. The human component is still fundamental and not all stages can be carried out digitally. However, it is expected that technical developments will rapidly lead to more and more digitalized therapies with an increase in the end quality of the therapy and less conditioned by the skills of the individual operator.

Author Contributions: Conceptualization, L.O.; methodology, L.O. and M.O.; software, L.O. and M.O.; resources, L.O.; data curation, F.G. and A.M.; writing—original draft preparation, L.O. and A.M.; writing—review and editing, L.O. and A.M.; visualization, L.O.; supervision, F.G.; M.O. fabricated the prosthesis. All authors have read and agreed to the published version of the manuscript.

Funding: This research received no external funding.

Acknowledgments: The authors thank Gianni Ortensi, Marco Ortensi, and Cesare Chiarini, who fabricated the prosthesis and supported laboratory digital processes.

Conflicts of Interest: The authors declare no conflict of interest.

References

1. Gupta, A.; Felton, D.A.; Jemt, T.; Koka, S. Rehabilitation of edentulism and mortality: A systematic review. *J. Prosthodont.* **2018**, *28*, 526–535. [CrossRef] [PubMed]
2. Kutkut, A.; Bertoli, E.; Frazer, R.; Pinto-Sinai, G.; Hidalgo, R.F.; Studts, J. A systematic review of studies comparing conventional complete denture and implant retained overdenture. *J. Prosthodont. Res.* **2018**, *62*, 1–9. [CrossRef] [PubMed]
3. Boven, G.C.; Raghoebar, G.; Vissink, A.; Meijer, H.J.A. Improving masticatory performance, bite force, nutritional state and patient's satisfaction with implant overdentures: A systematic review of the literature. *J. Oral Rehabil.* **2014**, *42*, 220–233. [CrossRef]
4. Schimmel, M.; Müller, F.; Suter, V.; Buser, D. Implants for elderly patients. *Periodontol. 2000* **2016**, *73*, 228–240. [CrossRef]
5. Ortensi, L.; Stefani, R.; Ortensi, G. Edentulous superior maxillary: Choosing the proper implant-supported prosthetic solution. *Spectr. Dialogue* **2015**, *14*, 3.

6. Tallarico, M.; Ortensi, L.; Martinolli, L.; Casucci, A.; Ferrari, E.; Malaguti, G.; Montanari, M.; Scrascia, R.; Vaccaro, G.; Venezia, P.; et al. Multicenter Retrospective Analysis of Implant Overdentures Delivered with Different Design and Attachment Systems: Results Between One and 17 Years of Follow-Up. *Dent. J.* **2018**, *6*, 71. [CrossRef]
7. Tallarico, M.; Cervino, G.; Scrascia, R.; Uccioli, U.; Lumbau, A.; Meloni, S.M. Minimally Invasive Treatment of Edentulous Maxillae with Overdenture Fully Supported by a Cad/Cam Titanium Bar with a Low-Profile Attachment Screwed on Four or Six Implants: A Case Series. *Prosthesis* **2020**, *2*, 6. [CrossRef]
8. Slot, W.; Raghoebar, G.M.; Cune, M.S.; Vissink, A.; Meijer, H.J. Maxillary overdentures supported by four or six implants in the anterior region: 5-year results from a randomized controlled trial. *J. Clin. Periodontol.* **2016**, *43*, 1180–1187. [CrossRef] [PubMed]
9. Coachman, C.C.; Calamita, M. Virtual Esthetic Smile Design. *J. Cosmet. Dent.* **2014**, *29*, 4.
10. Caviggioli, I.; Molinelli, F.; Ortensi, L.L.; Riccardo, S. La prima visita in odontoiatria protesica: Aspetti innovativi. *Il Dentista Moderno* **2011**, *6*, 46–54.
11. Lo Giudice, A.; Ortensi, L.; Farronato, M.; Lucchese, A.; Lo Castro, E.E.; Isola, G. The step further smile virtual planning: Milled versus prototyped mock-ups for the evaluation of the designed smile characteristics. *BMC Oral Health* **2020**, *20*, 165. [CrossRef] [PubMed]
12. Goodacre, C.J.; Garbacea, A.; Naylor, W.P.; Daher, T.; Marchack, C.B.B.; Lowry, J. CAD/CAM fabricated complete dentures: Concepts and clinical methods of obtaining required morphological data. *J. Prosthet. Dent.* **2012**, *107*, 34–46. [CrossRef]
13. Infante, L.; Yilmaz, B.; McGlumphy, E.E.; Finger, I. Fabricating complete dentures with CAD/CAM technology. *J. Prosthet. Dent.* **2014**, *111*, 351–355. [CrossRef]
14. Kattadiyil, M.T.; Jekki, R.; Goodacre, C.J.J.; Baba, N.Z. Comparison of treatment outcomes in digital and conventional complete removable dental prosthesis fabrications in a predoctoral setting. *J. Prosthet. Dent.* **2015**, *114*, 818–825. [CrossRef] [PubMed]
15. Tallarico, M.; Scrascia, R.; Annucci, M.; Meloni, S.; Lumbau, A.; Koshovari, A.; Xhanari, E.; Martinolli, M. Errors in Implant Positioning Due to Lack of Planning: A Clinical Case Report of New Prosthetic Materials and Solutions. *Materials* **2020**, *13*, 1883. [CrossRef] [PubMed]
16. Avrampou, M.; Mericske-Stern, R.; Blatz, M.B.; Katsoulis, J. Virtual implant planning in the edentulous maxilla: Criteria for decision making of prosthesis design. *Clin. Oral Implant. Res.* **2013**, *24*, 152–159. [CrossRef]
17. Ortensi, L.; Martini, M.; Montanari, M.; Galassini, G. A Simplified Method to Identify Patient Face Type for a Prosthodontic Treatment Plan. *J. Dent. Health Oral Disord. Ther.* **2017**, *8*, 1–5. [CrossRef]
18. Nishi, S.E.; Basri, R.; Alam, M.K. Uses of electromyography in dentistry: An overview with meta-analysis. *Eur. J. Dent.* **2016**, *10*, 419. [CrossRef]
19. Stefani, R.; Caviggioli, I.; Molinelli, F.; Ortensi, L. L'impiego delle tecnologie digitali nella diagnosi protesica e nella realizzazione della protesi. *Il Dentista Moderno* **2012**, *10*, 46–75.
20. McLaren, E.A.; Terry, D. Photography in dentistry. *J. Calif. Dent. Assoc.* **2001**, *29*, 735–742.
21. Ortensi, L.; Stefani, R.; Lavorgna, L.; Caviggioli, I.; Vitali, T. A Digital Workflow for an Implant Retained Overdenture: A New Approach. *Biomed. J. Sci. Tech. Res.* **2018**, *6*. [CrossRef]
22. D'Arienzo, L.F.; D'Arienzo, A.; Borracchini, A. Comparison of the suitability of intra-oral scanning with conventional impression of edentulous maxilla in vivo. A preliminary study. *J. Osseointegr.* **2018**, *10*, 115–120.
23. Bonato, G.; Borracchini, A.; Borromeo, C.; Capezzuto, V.; Casucci, A.; Chimenz, S.; Colognesi, R.; Colombo, M.; Gassino, G.; Ferrone, U.; et al. *Aspetti Clinico Tecnici Nella Protesi Combinata*; Teamwork Media srl: Brescia, Italy, 2015.
24. Joda, T.; Brägger, U.; Gallucci, G. Systematic literature review of digital three-dimensional superimposition techniques to create virtual dental patients. *Int. J. Oral Maxillofac. Implant.* **2015**, *30*, 330–337. [CrossRef]
25. Burkhardt, M.A.; Waser, J.; Milleret, V.; Gerber, I.; Emmert, M.; Foolen, J.; Hoerstrup, S.P.; Schlottig, F.; Vogel, V. Synergistic interactions of blood-borne immune cells, fibroblasts and extracellular matrix drive repair in an in vitro peri-implant wound healing model. *Sci. Rep.* **2016**, *6*, 21071. [CrossRef] [PubMed]
26. Scrascia, R.; Fiorillo, L.; Gaita, V.; Secondo, L.; Nicita, F.; Cervino, G. Implant-Supported Prosthesis for Edentulous Patient Rehabilitation. From Temporary Prosthesis to Definitive with a New Protocol: A Single Case Report. *Prosthesis* **2020**, *2*, 2. [CrossRef]

27. Lavorgna, L.; Vitali, T.; Caviggioli, I.; Ortensi, L. Fully Digital Workflow for an Implant Retained Overdenture by Digital Smile Project to Guided Surgery and Prosthetic Rehabilitation. *Int. J. Sci. Res.* **2018**, *7*, 12.
28. Ortensi, L.; Vitali, T.; Bonfiglioli, R.; Grande, F. New Tricks in the Preparation Design for Prosthetic Ceramic Laminate Veeners. *Prosthesis* **2019**, *1*, 5. [CrossRef]
29. Doundoulakis, J.H.; Eckert, S.E.; Lindquist, C.C.; Jeffcoat, M.K. The implant-supported overdenture as an alternative to the complete mandibular denture. *J. Am. Dent. Assoc.* **2003**, *134*, 1455–1458. [CrossRef] [PubMed]
30. Assunção, W.G.; Zardo, G.G.; Delben, J.A.; Barão, V.A. Comparing the efficacy of mandibular implant-retained overdentures and conventional dentures among elderly edentulous patients: Satisfaction and quality of life. *Gerodontology* **2007**, *24*, 235–238. [CrossRef]
31. Hamada, M.O.; Garrett, N.R.; Roumanas, E.D.; Kapur, K.K.; Freymiller, E.; Han, T.; Diener, R.M.; Chen, T.; Levin, S. A randomized clinical trial comparing the efficacy of mandibular implant-supported overdentures and conventional dentures in diabetic patients. Part IV: Comparisons of dietary intake. *J. Prosthet. Dent.* **2001**, *85*, 53–60. [CrossRef]
32. Jemt, T. Failures and complications in 391 consecutively inserted fixed prostheses supported by branemark implants in edentulous jaws: A study of treatment from the time of prosthesis placement to the first annual checkup. *Int. J. Oral Maxillofac. Implant.* **1991**, *6*, 270–276.
33. Lundqvist, S.; Lohmander, A.; Haraldson, T. Speech before and after treatment with bridges on osseointegrated implants in the edentulous upper jaw. *Clin. Oral Implant. Res.* **1992**, *3*, 57–62. [CrossRef] [PubMed]
34. Lavorgna, L.; Cervino, G.; Fiorillo, L.; Di Leo, G.; Troiano, G.; Ortensi, M.; Galantucci, L.; Cicciù, M. Reliability of a Virtual Prosthodontic Project Realized through a 2D and 3D Photographic Acquisition: An Experimental Study on the Accuracy of Different Digital Systems. *Int. J. Environ. Res. Public Health* **2019**, *16*, 5139. [CrossRef] [PubMed]

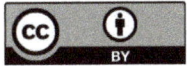

© 2020 by the authors. Licensee MDPI, Basel, Switzerland. This article is an open access article distributed under the terms and conditions of the Creative Commons Attribution (CC BY) license (http://creativecommons.org/licenses/by/4.0/).

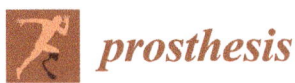

Article

Prevalence of Meibomian Gland Dysfunction and Its Effect on Quality of Life and Ocular Discomfort in Patients with Prosthetic Eyes

Alessandro Meduri [1,*], Rino Frisina [2], Miguel Rechichi [3] and Giovanni William Oliverio [1]

1. BIOMORF Deperatement, Ophthalmology Clinici, University of Messina, 98124 Messina, Italy; g.w89@me.com
2. Department of Ophthalmology, University of Padua, 35121 Padua, Italy; frisinarino@unipd.com
3. Centro Polispecialistico Mediterraneo, 88050 Sellia Marina, Italy; miguel.rechichi@libero.it
* Correspondence: ameduri@unime.it

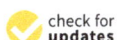

Received: 23 April 2020; Accepted: 8 June 2020; Published: 9 June 2020

Abstract: Purpose: To evaluate the influence of ocular discomfort and meibomian gland dysfunction (MGD) on quality of life in patients with an ocular prosthesis. Methods: a prospective analysis was conducted on 18 patients with a unilateral ocular prosthesis. Evaluation of ocular discomfort symptoms, lid margin abnormalities (LMA), meibomian gland expression, meibography and a psychometric evaluation using the National Eye Institute Visual Function Questionnaire (NEI VFQ), Facial Appearance subscale of the Negative Physical Self Scale (NPSS-F), Hospital Anxiety and Depression Scale (HADS) and the DAS24 to evaluate anxiety and depression. Results: the statistically significant differences observed between normal and prosthetic eyes related to ocular symptoms and the meibography score ($p = 0.0003$). A negative correlation was reported between NEI VFQ score and meibography score ($r = -0.509$; p-value $= 0.022$). A positive correlation was detected with NPSS ($r = 0.75$; p-value < 0.0001), anxiety HADS score ($r = 0.912$; p-value $= 0.001$) and depression HADS score ($r = 0.870$; p-value > 0.0001). Conclusion: MGD represents the most common cause of evaporative dry eye disease, due to the reduction of the thickness of the lipid layer of the tear film. The occurrence of MGD in patients with prosthetic eyes is very common. Anxiety and depression were correlated to ocular discomfort and MGD, and this could affect the quality of life in patients with an ocular prosthesis.

Keywords: ocular prosthesis; meibomian gland dysfunction; quality of life; ocular discomfort

1. Introduction

The loss of an eye presents severe emotional stress and commonly results in negative consequences to social behavior. Patients with an ocular prosthesis reported a high level of anxiety and depression as a consequence of their changed appearance. In this sense, the use of an ocular prosthesis purposes to improve cosmetic appearance, as well as ameliorating social acceptance [1]. Nowadays, ocular prosthesis can be stock or patient-customized, considering several factors, such as the anatomy and tissue bed of the socket, and individualized aesthetic requirements. The main material used for the fabrication of ocular prostheses is polymethyl methacrylate (PMMA), which is compatible with tissues, and has easy color modification abilities and elevated aesthetic appearance. Numerous techniques to improve the aesthetic results of the ocular prosthesis have been proposed, such as painting the sclera and iris, the use of transparent grids for proper orientation and the use of a digital image of the normal eye [2]. The principal causes for the need of an ocular prosthesis comprise tumors, congenital defects and malformations, irreparable trauma, end-stage eye diseases, and severe ocular diseases associated with uncontrolled pain, such as neovascular glaucoma, or an unattractive appearance, such as phthisis bulbi [3,4]. Eye removal surgery is classified into evisceration, enucleation and exenteration. Evisceration includes the removal of the ocular contents, leaving in place the sclera shell. The mobility of the eviscerated globe implant is preserved, since the extraocular muscles are intact. Enucleation consists in the removal of the eyeball after the extraocular muscles and the optic nerve have been separated. Sufficient space is formed for the prosthesis, with movement of the fornix within the enucleated socket providing mobility to the ocular prosthesis. Exenteration is the surgical removal of the complete contents of the orbit. The eyelids may or may not be involved. Exenteration defects in some instances may be allowed to heal by secondary intent, but adequate space must remain in the resultant defect to allow the prosthesis to be positioned superiorly and posteriorly enough for a good cosmetic appearance [5]. An orbital implant is used to fill the orbital cavity or the scleral shell, and to replace the consequent volume reduction due to the removal of the eye. The eye's motility is preserved, as the scleral implant is attached to the ocular muscles. Several types of implants exist, differing in shape (spherical or oval), being stock or customized, porous or non-porous, and in the presence of a peg or motility post [4,5]. Chronic ocular discomfort represents one of the most common adverse events referred to in long-standing patients with an ocular prosthesis. Many patients with an ocular prosthesis report varying degrees of ocular discomfort, such as discharge, dryness, irritation and a sticky sensation. Numerous mechanisms that could lead to ocular discomfort in prosthetic eye wearers were suggested, such as the infection of the anophthalmic socket, glutinous surface deposits and a roughened prosthesis [6,7]. A recent study analyzed the role of the tear film and demonstrated the linear correlation between tear deficiency and discomfort reported in patients with an ocular prosthesis [7]. Recent studies also confirmed the relationship between MGD and contact lens wear, as well as in ocular prosthesis wear, demonstrating a larger grade of Meibomian gland loss and alterations compared with normal paired eyelids [8,9]. Meibomian gland dysfunction (MGD) represents the most common cause of evaporative dry eye disease, due to the reduction of the thickness of the lipid layer of the tear film [10]. The aim of this study is to evaluate the prevalence of MGD in patients with ocular prostheses reporting symptoms of ocular discomfort, and their impact on quality of life.

2. Results

Demographic data is reported in Table 1. Eighteen patients of mean age 51.3 ± 16.8 years and mean length of prosthesis duration 13.6 ± 5.1 years were studied. The most frequent causes of blindness were trauma (ten patients), cancer (five patients) and other ocular diseases (three patients) such as endophthalmitis and one case of neo-vascular glaucoma. A case of unilateral ocular prosthesis due to neo-vascular glaucoma is reported in Figure 1. Evisceration was the most common surgery (10 patients). All ocular prostheses were polymethyl methacrylate (PMMA). Sixteen patients had a customized prosthesis, presenting a good aesthetic appearance. Only two patients had a stock prosthesis. In Table 2 summarises scores regarding ocular symptoms, lid margin abnormalities (LMA), meibomian gland expression and meiboscore related to the normal eye and the prosthetic eye in the upper and lower eyelid. Significant statistical differences were noted between the normal eye and prosthetic eye related to ocular symptoms (p-value < 0.0001), LMA (p = 0.0006), meibomian gland expression score (p = 0.0003), and in the meiboscore of the upper eyelid (p = 0.0004), lower eyelid (p = 0.0003) and total meiboscore (p = 0.0003). A positive correlation between duration of prosthesis and meiboscore in the prosthetic eye r = 0.878; p < 0.001 95% CI: [0.688, 0.956] was observed. All psychometric data are reported in Table 3. A negative correlation was reported between NEI VFQ score and meiboscore (r = −0.509; p-value = 0.022). Positive correlations were detected with NPSS (r = 0.75; p-value < 0.0001); anxiety HADS score (r = 0.912; p-value < 0.001); depression HADS score (r = 0.870; p-value < 0.0001); DES24 (r = 0.686; p-value < 0.0001) and VAS score for sadness (r = 0.657; p-value = 0.002) anger (r = 0.741; p-value < 0.0001) and shamefulness (r = 0.744; p-value < 0.0001). (Figure 2 and Table 4).

Table 1. Clinical Characteristics of the Study Population.

Parameters	Value
Total patients	18
Age (years)	51.3 ± 16.8
Gender	
Male	10 (55.6%)
Female	8 (44.4%)
Duration of prosthesis (years)	13.6 ± 5.1
Cause of eye loss	
Trauma	10 (55.6%)
Cancer	5 (27.8%)
Further disease	3 (16.6%)
Surgery	
Evisceration	10 (55.6%)
Enucleation	8 (44.4%)

Data are presented as n (%), and mean ± standard deviation.

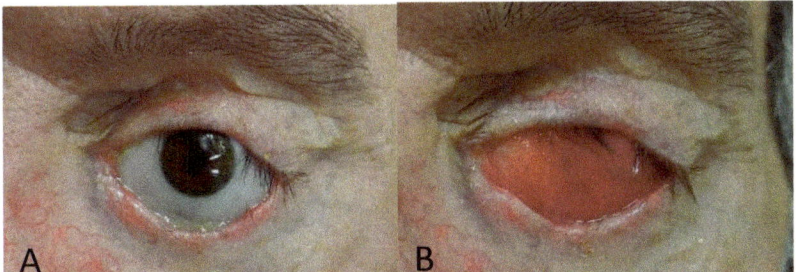

Figure 1. Ocular prosthesis (**A**), anophthalmic socket (**B**).

Table 2. Comparison of meibomian gland and lid margin evaluation in prosthesis and normal eye.

	Prosthetic Eye (Mean ± SD)	Normal Eye (Mean ± SD)	p-Value *
Symptoms score	8.8 ± 2.8	2.5 ± 1.7	**<0.0001**
Lid margin abnormalities	2.1 ± 0.7	0.4 ± 0.6	**0.0006**
Meibomian gland expression	2.5 ± 0.6	0.4 ± 0.5	**0.0003**
Meiboscore			
Upper eyelid	2 ± 0.7	0.4 ± 0.5	**0.0004**
Lower eyelid	1.3 ± 0.5	0.2 ± 0.4	**0.0003**
Complessive	3.1 ± 0.78	0.41 ± 0.5	**0.0003**

All data are reported as mean ± standard deviation. * Wilcoxon signed-rank test. Bold characters for p-value < 0.05.

Table 3. Psychometric data.

	Score (Mean ± SD)
Vision-specific composite	38.4 ± 16.9
Appearance concern	2.8 ± 1.13
Shame	4.94 ± 2.33
Sadness	5.35 ± 2.87
Anger	5.52 ± 2.15
Anxiety	6.76 ± 2.33
Depression	6.29 ± 2.77
DAS24	45.88 ± 25.63

Vision-specific composite refers to NEI VFQ score; appearance concern refers to NPSS score; shame, sadness and anger were evaluated using a visual analogue score. All data are reported as mean ± standard deviation.

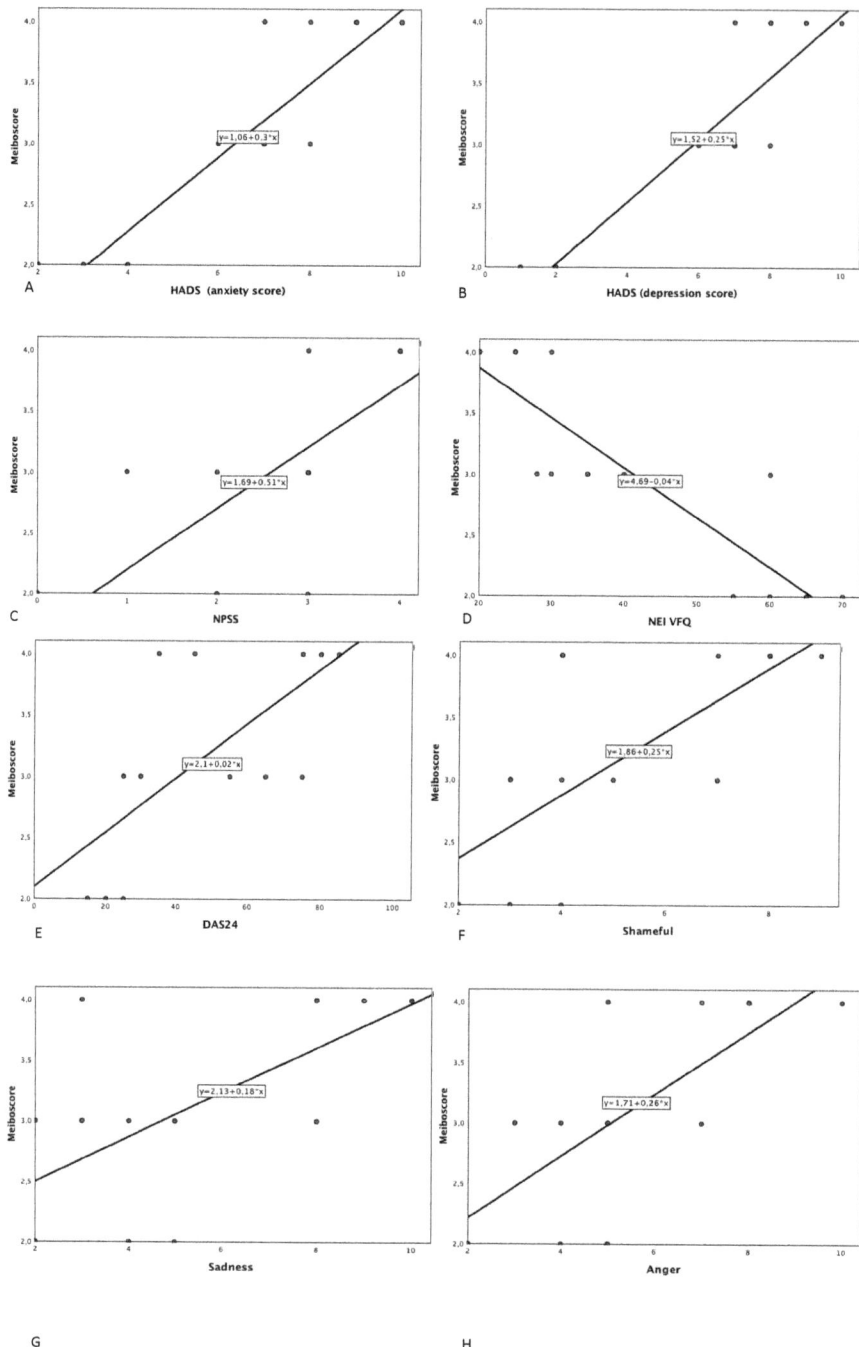

Figure 2. Scatter plot showing the relationship between total meiboscore (total) and (**A**) Hospital Anxiety and Depression Scale (anxiety score); (**B**) Hospital Anxiety and Depression Scale (depression score); (**C**) Negative Physical Self Scale-Facial appearance subscale score; (**D**) National Eye Institute Visual Function Questionnaire; (**E**) Derriford Appearance Scale; (**F**) Shameful (visual analogue scale); (**G**) Sadness (visual analogue scale); (**H**) Anger (visual analogue scale).

Table 4. Pearson's correlation between Meiboscore (total) and psychometric score.

	r	p-Value *
NEI VFQ	−0.884	<0.001
NPSS	0.732	<0.001
HADS (Anxiety)	0.912	<0.001
HADS (Depression)	0.870	<0.001
DAS24	0.686	<0.001
Shameful	0.744	<0.001
Sadness	0.657	0.002
Anger	0.741	<0.001

Legend: NEI VFQ—The National Eye Institute Visual Function Questionnaire; NPSS-Negative Physical Self Scale; HADS—Hospital Anxiety and Depression Scale; DAS-24—Derriford Appearance Scale.* ANOVA test, bold characters for p-value < 0.05.

3. Discussion

Chronic ocular discomfort represents one of the most common adverse events referred to in long-standing patients with an ocular prosthesis. Chronic discharge, in patients with an ocular prosthesis, could be related to several conditions. In particular, they could be classified as prosthesis-related, such as poor fit, mechanical irritation, reaction to deposits and poor prosthesis hygiene; socket and implant-related, such as exposure, granuloma, peg-related, socket contraction and environmental allergens; lacrimal-related, such as reduced tear production or outflow obstruction; or eyelid-related, such as MGD, lagophthalmos and lack of mucous membrane or skin. A common condition of ocular discomfort in a long-standing patient with ocular prosthesis is giant papillary conjunctivitis, due to a prolonged mechanical irritation and the immunologic reaction of the ocular surface [11,12]. Rokohl et al. documented a relationship between the discharge severity of prosthetic eyewear with conjunctival inflammation, higher cleaning frequency and less hand washing before handling [13]. The role of reduced tear production was documented in previous studies. A reduced tear volume was documented in anophthalmic patients, as demonstrated by a reduced Schirmer's test value, as well as a low tear meniscus height [14,15].

Recent studies have also considered the morphologic changes in meibomian glands related to prosthetic eye patients, demonstrating a larger grade of meibomian gland loss compared with the normal paired eyelids [8,9]. In the present study, a high prevalence of MGD was recognized in the population of patients evaluated. In particular, significant differences were demonstrated between the normal eye and the prosthetic eye, concerning ocular symptoms (p-value > 0.0001), LMA (p = 0.0006), meibomian gland expression score (p = 0.0003), lid margin abnormalities (p = 0.0006) and meiboscore (p = 0.0003). Meiboscore was evaluated using Keratograph 5M (Oculus, Wetzlar, Germany) to acquire a noninvasive meibography. MGD describes a group of disorders characterized by functional abnormalities of the meibomian glands. The International Workshop defined MGD a chronic, diffuse abnormality of the meibomian glands, commonly characterized by terminal duct obstruction and/or qualitative/quantitative changes in glandular secretion [16]. MGD can lead to altered tear film composition, ocular surface disease, ocular and eyelid discomfort, and evaporative dry eye. In fact, MGD represents the principal cause of evaporative dry eye [17]. Eyelids of a prosthetic eye seem mostly disposed to obstructive MGD, as result of an increased hyperkeratinization, causing excretory duct obstruction, due to a combination of tear deficiency, deposit accumulation, and micro-trauma. Other hypothetical pathophysiological mechanisms of meibomian gland obstruction, in the eyelid of patients with an ocular prosthesis, is decreased and weakened eyelid blinking. Recently, it was suggested that tear insufficiency as consequent of MGD may be the cause of ocular discomfort for those patients, particularly in whom no specific etiology can be identified. Dry eye symptoms are common in long-standing ocular prosthesis wearers. In this study, a significant difference was demonstrated by comparing the normal eye and prosthetic eye (p-value < 0.0001) relative to ocular discomfort symptoms. Duration of the prosthesis may play a central role; thus, a positive correlation with meiboscore in prosthetic eye was seen (r = 0.878, $p < 0.001$). Jang, et al. reported a greater degree of meibomian gland loss in patients who had used an ocular prosthesis longer than 10 years. In our group of patients, the average duration of prosthesis use was 13.6 ± 5.1 years. For this reason, MGD could represent an undiagnosed cause of chronic ocular discomfort in long-standing ocular prosthesis patients. The occurrence of biofilm growth has been confirmed on many ocular prostheses. Biofilms may play a significant role in the tolerability of the ocular prosthesis. However, biofilm has also been identified on the surface of scleral implants, without signs of clinical infection. The longstanding ocular prosthesis has been related to the development of giant papillary conjunctivitis, resulting in poor tolerability [18]. Litwin, et al. analyzed the role of the degree of prosthesis surface polishing, comparing the standard and the optical polishing procedures. They reported better tolerability at 12 months in the optical polish of the prosthesis group [19]. Patients with an ocular prosthesis reported a high level of social anxiety, and avoid social situations as a consequence of their altered appearance. This was documented by the mean score (2.8 ± 1.13) relative to the Facial Appearance subscale of the Negative Physical Self Scale (NPSS). A score > 2 was observed in eight patients, indicating displeasure with facial appearance. Similar results were also noted relative to the DAS24 questionnaire score. The mean score of DAS24 in our group of patients was 45.88 ± 25.63.

DAS24 is a measure of social anxiety and social avoidance in relation to appearance. Sixteen patients had a customized prosthesis, presenting a good aesthetic appearance.

The lowest questionnaire scores were found only in the two patients with stock prostheses.

The HADS is a psychometrical scale assessing patients' anxiety and depression levels related to health problems. Considering the score of the HADS questionnaire, a high level of depression (6.29 ± 2.77) and anxiety (6.76 ± 2.33) were detected in our population of patients.

Chronic ocular discomfort could represent a factor that increases the anxiety condition, in patients with an altered appearance. Several studies have shown an association of dry eye disease with depression and anxiety. However, a direct correlation between the severity of dry eye disease and anxiety or depression was not demonstrated [20]. It is plausible to consider an increased risk of developing anxious and depressive disorders in patients with an ocular prosthesis with symptoms of dry eye and MGD. In fact, a higher score of anxiety and depression was recognized in patients presenting symptoms and signs of MGD. In particular, a statistically significant direct correlation was observed between meiboscore and the anxiety HADS score (r = 0.912; p-value = 0.001), as well as with the depression HADS score (r = 0.870; p-value > 0.0001 (Figure 2)).

Nevertheless, several factors could influence the psychological behavior of patients, and a chronic ocular discomfort could represent a single factor inside a wide variety of causes. In conclusion, this study suggests that anxiety and depression conditions could be common in patients with eye prostheses, in particular in the presence of chronic ocular discomfort caused by MGD. This result should be confirmed in a bigger cohort of patients, to find other factors, such as sex, age, therapy and metabolic differences, that could play a direct influence.

4. Materials and Methods

A prospective, multi-centric analysis was conducted on 18 patients (ten male, eight female) with a unilateral ocular prosthesis, between July 2018 and January 2020. The study was conducted in accordance with the tenets of the Declaration of Helsinki. All patients signed an informed consent after a full explanation of all study-related procedures. Inclusion criteria were ability and willingness to participate in the study, unilateral ocular prosthesis worn at least 2 years and subjective symptoms and signs of ocular discomfort such as burning, wetness, foreign body sensation, pain, itching, dryness, tearing and mucous discharge. Patients with inflammation or infection of the socket, or with a poorly fitted prosthesis were excluded from the study. Each patient was questioned about their duration of prosthesis use and the type of ophthalmic surgery (such as evisceration or enucleation) requiring ocular prosthesis.

4.1. Symptom Evaluation

Patients were asked to assign severity using this scale for the following symptoms: burning, wetness, foreign body sensation, pain, itching, dryness, tearing, mucous discharge, hyperemia, excessive blinking, uncomfortable in windy conditions and uncomfortable in dry conditions, evaluated according to a scoring system from 0 (absent) to 3 (severe). A global score was obtained by summing up the scores of each symptom and the values (score range 0–36). The assessment of symptoms was the same for the prosthetic eye-wearing side and for the normal side.

4.2. Meibomian Gland and Lid Margin Evaluation

A slit-lamp examination was conducted to evaluate lid margin abnormalities and meibomian gland expression. Lid margin abnormalities were scored from 0 to 4 based on the presence or absence of the following parameters: irregular lid margin, plugging of meibomian gland orifices, vascular engorgement, or a shift in the mucocutaneous junction [10]. Meibomian gland expression was assigned grades for clarity and ease of meibum expression (grade 1–4). Meibography was performed using a Keratograph 5M (Oculus, Wetzlar, Germany) in the upper and lower eyelid separately. Meiboscore grading was assessed by Keratograph 5M automatic software (JENVIS Meibo Grading Scales). Grade 0: no loss of Meibomian glands; Grade 1: loss of less than 1/3 of the total meibomian gland area; Grade 2: loss of 1/3 to 2/3 of the total area; Grade 3: loss of more than 2/3 of the area. The total Meiboscore was considered as the sum of the meiboscore of the upper eyelid and lower eyelid [21].

4.3. Psychosocial Variables

Four standardized questionnaires assessing quality of life, anxiety and depression related to physical health problems, social anxiety and social avoidance in relation to appearance, and three supplementary elements examining the level of shamefulness, sadness and anger felt using a visual analogue scale (0–10). The National Eye Institute Visual Function Questionnaire (NEI VFQ) is a questionnaire assessing the quality of life related to visual function, comprising several subcategories including general and peripheral vision, color perception, ocular discomfort, near and distance activities, social performance, mental healthiness and driving ability. A complex score is estimated by the average of the subcategories' scores (0–100). Lower scores denote poor functioning [22]. The Facial Appearance subscale of the Negative Physical Self Scale (NPSS) is an effective measure of appearance, comprising five categories. We considered the Facial Appearance subscale. The NPSS-F score is estimated by the average of the item scores (>2 indicating displeasure with facial appearance) [23]. The Hospital Anxiety and Depression Scale (HADS) was used to evaluate the level of anxiety and depression. The HADS comprises seven items (scored 0–3) about anxiety, and seven items about depression (scored 0–3). Total scores range from 0 to 21 for both subcategories, with lower scores signifying low levels of anxiety or depression [24]. The DAS24 is a measure of social anxiety and social avoidance in relation to appearance. The total score ranges from 11 to 96, with high scores signifying high levels of social anxiety and social avoidance [25].

4.4. Statistical Analysis

The numerical data were expressed as mean and standard deviation, and the categorical variables as absolute frequency and percentage. Examined variables did not present normal distribution, as verified by the Kolmogorov Smirnov test; consequently, the non-parametric approach was used. For each parameter, we performed statistical comparisons between the normal eye and the prosthetic eye in the exam, using the Wilcoxon signed-rank test for numerical variables. The Pearson correlation coefficient (r) was calculated to measure the strength of correlations between parameters. Statistical analyses were performed using JASP (Version 0.11.1). A p-value smaller than 0.05 was considered to be statistically significant.

Author Contributions: Conceptualization, G.W.O. and A.M.; methodology, G.W.O.; software, G.W.O.; validation, A.M., R.F. and M.R.; formal analysis, G.W.O.; investigation, A.M.; resources, A.M.; data curation, G.W.O.; writing—original draft preparation, G.W.O.; writing—review and editing, A.M.; visualization, R.M.; supervision, A.M.; project administration, A.M.; funding acquisition, A.M. All authors have read and agreed to the published version of the manuscript.

Funding: This research received no external funding.

Conflicts of Interest: The authors declare no conflict of interest.

References

1. McBain, H.B.; Ezra, D.G.; Rose, G.E.; Newman, S.P.; Appearance Research Collaboration (ARC). The psychosocial impact of living with an ocular prosthesis. *Orbit* **2013**, *33*, 39–44. [CrossRef] [PubMed]
2. Kulkarni, R.S.; Kulkarni, P.; Shah, R.J.; Tomar, B. Aesthetically Characterized Ocular Prosthesis. *J. Coll. Physicians Surg. Pak.* **2018**, *28*, 476–478. [CrossRef] [PubMed]
3. Modugno, A.; Mantelli, F.; Sposato, S.; Moretti, C.; Lambiase, A.; Bonini, S. Ocular prostheses in the last century: A retrospective analysis of 8018 patients. *Eye* **2013**, *27*, 865–870. [CrossRef] [PubMed]
4. Zigiotti, G.L.; Cavarretta, S.; Morara, M.; Nam, S.M.; Ranno, S.; Pichi, F.; Lembo, A.; Lupo, S.; Nucci, P.; Meduri, A. Standard enucleation with aluminium oxide implant (bioceramic) covered with patient's sclera. *Sci. World J.* **2012**, *2012*, 481584. [CrossRef]
5. Sajjad, A. Ocular Prosthesis—A Simulation of Human Anatomy: A Literature Review. *Cureus* **2012**, *4*, e74. [CrossRef]
6. Jones, C.A.; Collin, J.R. A classification and review the causes of discharging sockets. *Trans. Ophthalmol. Soc. UK* **1983**, *103*, 351–353.
7. Malhotra, R. Ocular prostheses: Not quite an eye for an eye. *Br. J. Ophthalmol.* **2013**, *97*, 383–385. [CrossRef]
8. Altin, M.E.; Karadeniz, S.U.; Kahraman, H.G. Meibomian Gland Dysfunction and Its Association with Ocular Discomfort in Patients with Ocular Prosthesis. *Eye Contact Lens* **2019**. [CrossRef]
9. Jang, S.Y.; Lee, S.Y.; Yoon, J.S. Meibomian gland dysfunction in longstanding prosthetic eye wearers. *Br. J. Ophthalmol.* **2013**, *97*, 398–402, Erratum in **2013**, *97*, 1362. [CrossRef]
10. Arita, R.; Itoh, K.; Maeda, S.; Maeda, K.; Furuta, A.; Fukuoka, S.; Tomidokoro, A.; Amano, S. Proposed Diagnostic Criteria for Obstructive Meibomian Gland Dysfunction. *Ophthalmology* **2009**, *116*, 2058–2063. [CrossRef]
11. Chang, W.J.; Tse, D.T.; Rosa, R.H.; Huang, A.J.W.; Johnson, T.E.; Schiffman, J. Conjunctival Cytology Features of Giant Papillary Conjunctivitis Associated with Ocular Prostheses. *Ophthalmic Plast. Reconstr. Surg.* **2005**, *21*, 39–45. [CrossRef] [PubMed]
12. Kim, J.H.; Lee, M.J.; Choung, H.K.; Kim, N.J.; Hwang, S.W.; Sung, M.S.; Khwarg, S.I. Conjunctival cytologic features in anophthalmic patients wearing an ocular prosthesis. *Ophthalmic Plast. Reconstr. Surg.* **2008**, *24*, 290–295. [CrossRef]
13. Rokohl, A.C.; Adler, W.; Koch, K.R.; Mor, J.M.; Jia, R.; Trester, M.; Pine, N.S.; Pine, K.R.; Heindl, L.M. Cryolite glass prosthetic eyes—The response of the anophthalmic socket. *Graefe's Arch. Clin. Exp. Ophthalmol.* **2019**, *257*, 2015–2023. [CrossRef] [PubMed]
14. Kim, S.E.; Yoon, J.S.; Lee, S.Y. Tear measurement in prosthetic eye users with fourier-domain optical coherence tomography. *Am. J. Ophthalmol.* **2010**, *149*, 602–607. [CrossRef] [PubMed]
15. Allen, L.; Kolder, H.E.; Bulgarelli, E.M.; Bulgarelli, D.M. Artificial eyes and tear measurements. *Ophthalmology* **1980**, *87*, 155–157. [CrossRef]
16. Nichols, K.K. The international workshop on meibomian gland dysfunction: Introduction. *Investig. Ophthalmol. Vis. Sci.* **2011**, *52*, 1917–1921. [CrossRef]
17. Chhadva, P.; Goldhardt, R.; Galor, A. Meibomian Gland Disease: The Role of Gland Dysfunction in Dry Eye Disease. *Ophthalmology* **2017**, *124*, S20–S26. [CrossRef]
18. Sun, M.T.; Pirbhai, A.; Selva, D. Bacterial biofilms associated with ocular prostheses. *Clin. Exp. Ophthalmol.* **2015**, *43*, 602–603. [CrossRef]
19. Litwin, A.S.; Worrell, E.; Roos, J.C.P.; Edwards, B.; Malhotra, R. Can We Improve the Tolerance of an Ocular Prosthesis by Enhancing Its Surface Finish? *Ophthalmic Plast. Reconstr. Surg.* **2018**, *34*, 130–135. [CrossRef]

20. Kaiser, T.; Janssen, B.; Schrader, S.; Geerling, G. Depressive symptoms, resilience, and personality traits in dry eye disease. *Graefe's Arch. Clin. Exp. Ophthalmol.* **2019**, *257*, 591–599. [CrossRef]
21. Pult, H.; Riede-Pult, B. Comparison of subjective grading and objective assessment in meibography. *Contact Lens Anterior Eye* **2013**, *36*, 22–27. [CrossRef] [PubMed]
22. Mangione, C.M.; Lee, P.P.; Gutierrez, P.R.; Spritzer, K.; Berry, S.; Hays, R.D. Development of the 25-item National Eye Institute Visual Function Questionnaire. *Arch. Ophthalmol.* **2001**, *119*, 1050–1058. [CrossRef]
23. Chen, H.; Jackson, T.; Huang, X. The Negative Physical Self Scale: Initial development and validation in samples of Chinese adolescents and young adults. *Body Image* **2006**, *3*, 401–412. [CrossRef] [PubMed]
24. Zigmond, A.S.; Snaith, R.P. The hospital anxiety and depression scale. *Acta Psychiatr. Scand.* **1983**, *67*, 361–370. [CrossRef] [PubMed]
25. Carr, T.; Harris, D.; James, C. The Derriford Appearance Scale (DAS-59): A new scale to measure individual responses to living with problems of appearance. *Br. J. Health Psychol.* **2000**, *5*, 201–215. [CrossRef]

© 2020 by the authors. Licensee MDPI, Basel, Switzerland. This article is an open access article distributed under the terms and conditions of the Creative Commons Attribution (CC BY) license (http://creativecommons.org/licenses/by/4.0/).

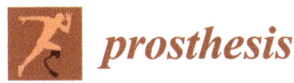

Article

A Finite Element Model for Trigger Finger

Helena I. Relf [1], Carla G. Barberio [2] and Daniel M. Espino [1,*]

1. Department of Mechanical Engineering, University of Birmingham, Birmingham B15 2TT, UK; H.I.Relf@bham.ac.uk
2. Walsall Manor Hospital, Walsall WS2 9PS, UK; carlabarberio@gmail.com
* Correspondence: d.m.espino@bham.ac.uk; Tel.: +44-(0)121-414-7355

Received: 12 June 2020; Accepted: 20 July 2020; Published: 22 July 2020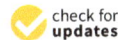

Abstract: The aim of this study was to develop a finite element model to investigate the forces on tendons which ensue due to trigger finger. The model was used to simulate both flexor and extensor tendons within the index finger; two test cases were defined, simulating a "mildly" and "severely" affected tendon by applying constraints. The finger was simulated in three different directions: extension, abduction and hyper-extension. There was increased tension during hyper-extension, with tension in the mildly affected tendon increasing from 1.54 to 2.67 N. Furthermore, there was a consistent relationship between force and displacement, with a substantial change in the gradient of the force when the constraints of the condition were applied for all movements. The intention of this study is that the simulation framework is used to enable the in silico development of novel prosthetic devices to aid with treatment of trigger finger, given that, currently, the non-surgical first line of treatment is a splint.

Keywords: biomechanics; finite element; hyper-extension; trigger finger; stenosing tenosynovitis; tendon; tension

1. Introduction

The hand is considered the most dexterous and well-coordinated part of the body, having great complexity and utility [1,2]. Its mobility is vital for any individual's independence during daily activities. Stenosing tenosynovitis, more commonly known as trigger finger, is one of the most common pathologies seen in hand surgery [3–5]. In a healthy hand, the flexor tendon should be able to move freely inside the tendon sheath. However, in this condition, the tendon and/or sheath become inflamed or irritated, forming scar tissue due to fibrocartilagenous metaplasia of the tendon, which restricts tendon movement through the sheath [6,7].

This restriction from trigger finger can result in painful locking and clicking of the finger [3,5,8–10]. "Triggering" refers to the sudden release of the tendon after catching during finger extension. Trigger finger is more commonly found in healthy middle-aged women [4,8,10,11] but is also associated with conditions such as diabetes, arthritis [10–13] and carpal tunnel syndrome [5,13]. The exact cause of the condition is unclear and can vary between cases, but the tendon can be further aggravated by hand use at work or during sport [12]. Symptoms include tenderness in the affected area, movement pain and locking or clicking; if attended to promptly, pain and swelling can be reduced easily. Surgery is only considered if other treatment options fail or the condition goes untreated for an extended period of time [8]. Non-surgical treatments include splinting, physiotherapy, nonsteroidal anti-inflammatory drugs and corticosteroid injections [3,8,10,12]. Surgery is performed under local anaesthetic, with an incision created in the roof of the tendon sheath in order to widen the tunnel so that the tendon can move freely [14].

The hand is comprised of twenty-seven different bones consisting of phalanges, metacarpals and carpals (Figure 1). Effective function is coordinated by a linkage system of tendons, ligaments and muscles. Tendons transmit loads from the bones to the intrinsic muscles and are interconnected by aponeuroses; this is commonly referred to as the extensor mechanism [15,16]. All fingers have an extensor tendon, located on the posterior surface of the hand, and two flexor tendons, located on the palmar side; furthermore, the second and fifth fingers have an additional extensor tendon. The extensor digitorum communis (EDC) straightens the finger [17] from both the proximal and distal interphalangeal joints. Flexing (bending) of the finger is achieved through the flexor digitorum profundus (FDP) and the flexor digitorum superficialis (FDS) tendons that connect to the distal and middle phalanx, respectively. Flexor tendons are channelled through and constricted by the tendon sheath [18], with some lubrication provided by synovial fluid.

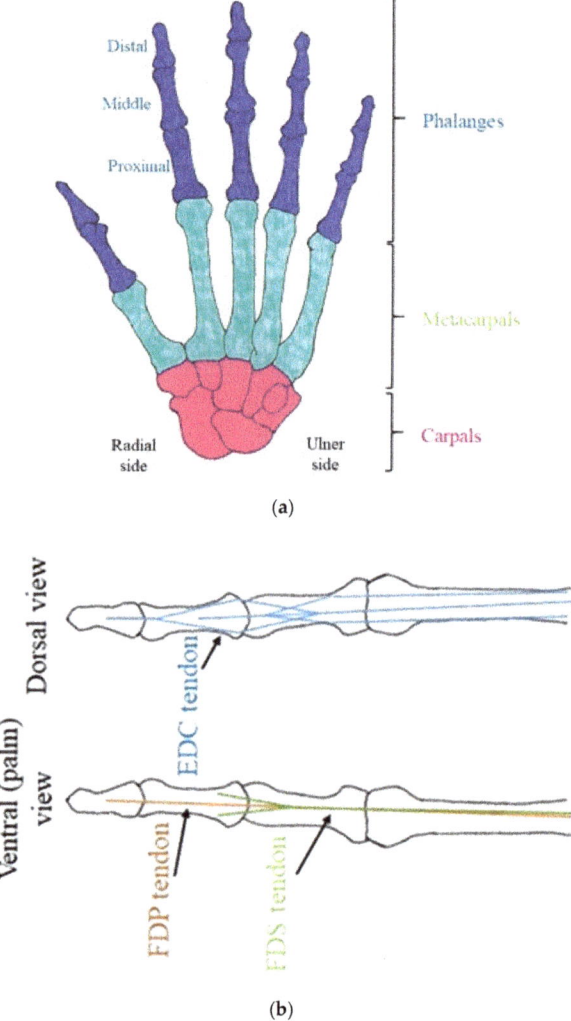

Figure 1. Schematic diagram of the hand. (**a**) Arrangement of the bones in the hand. (**b**) Simplified diagram of the attachment point of tendons in a finger.

There is limited research on the biomechanical impact of trigger finger and how it immobilises and generates stress within the hand. Most existing studies have been based on physical examinations of patients with the condition, using methods such as motion analysis and electromagnetic tracking systems. The higher the grade, the lower the range of movement for each joint in the finger, and restricted tendon mobility can measurably change comparative exerted force between the thumb and fingers [19,20]. Long-term, however, even after treatment, some disability may persist [21]. While a few biomechanical models are available for determining forces in tendons of the hand, limitations persist for their extrapolation to an understanding of the mechanics of trigger finger. For example, some models are specific to climbing techniques [22]. Others explore the finger extensor tendon network but do not model trigger finger [2]. Arguably, the most comprehensive model is provided by Lu et al. [23] to evaluate the forces within different tendons, predicting higher tension in the FDP tendon than in the FDS tendon when both tendons were triggering. There is scope, though, to evaluate the effect of trigger finger on the tension in the tendons of the hand during a range of movements. Such a model would enable a simulation framework to be available to test future prosthetic devices intended to aid in trigger finger "treatment", as an objective technique for early stage development.

The aim of this study is to develop a model, using finite element analysis (FEA), which can predict the forces within tendons in the hand during trigger finger. The focus is on the right hand's index finger as this is where trigger finger is most likely to occur [14]. Models developed include a healthy case along with both a mild and a severe model for trigger finger to enable direct comparison. The contribution made by this study is, therefore, in developing an FEA model for mild and severe levels of stenosing tenosynovitis (i.e., trigger finger).

2. Results

2.1. Outline of Results

Figures 2–8 present the results for the forces acting on the tendons and their displacement. Stress–strain curves have also been plotted to analyse the data. Forces on the tendons followed a nonlinear relationship, with clear differences between healthy tendons and those with the constraints of mild and severe trigger finger. The effects of extension, abduction and hyper-extension are outlined in Sections 2.2–2.4, with Section 2.5 outlining the variation of tension and cross-sectional area within a tendon.

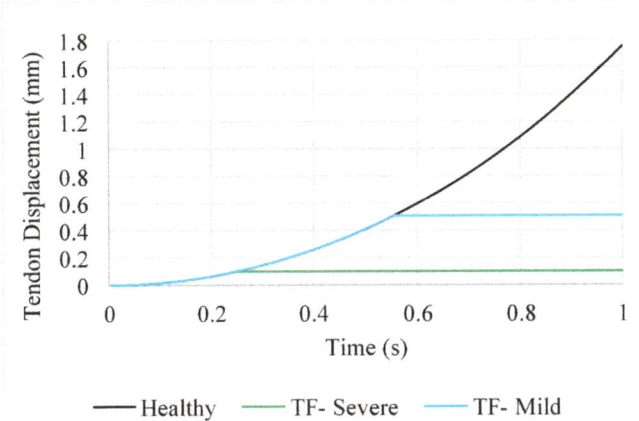

Figure 2. Tendon displacement for position A for healthy, mildly and severely affected tendons.

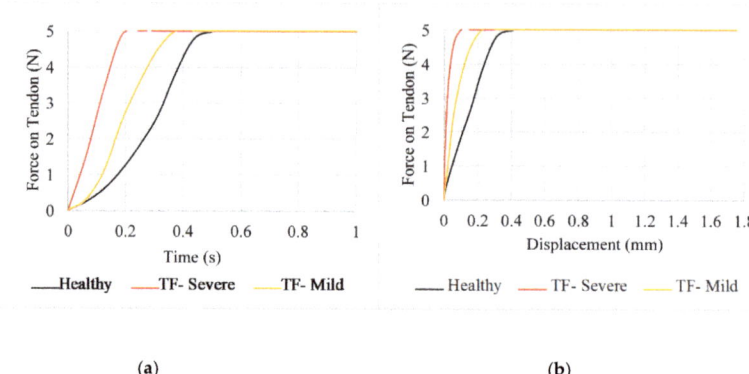

Figure 3. Force predicted for flexor digitorum profundus (FDP) and flexor digitorum superficialis (FDS) tendons (position A). (**a**) Force against time for the FDP and FDS tendons, (**b**) force against displacement of the FDP and FDS tendons.

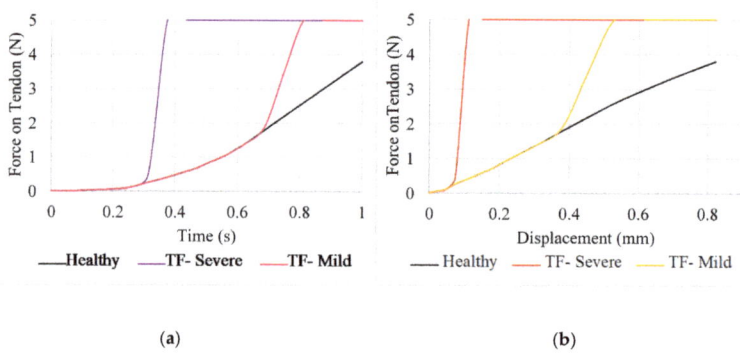

Figure 4. Force predicted for the extensor digitorum communis (EDC) tendon (position A). (**a**) Force against time, (**b**) force against displacement.

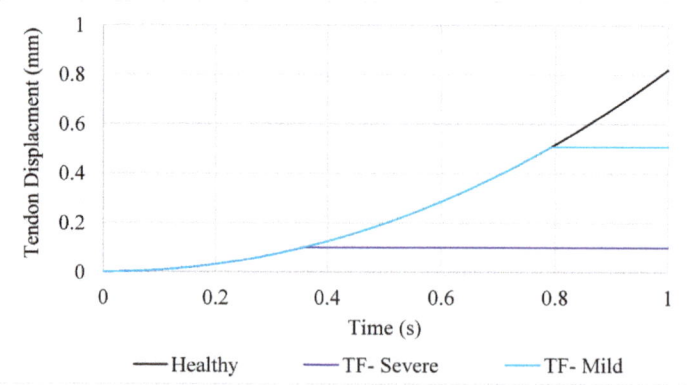

Figure 5. Time-dependent displacement of the FDS tendon (position A; note: TF: trigger finger).

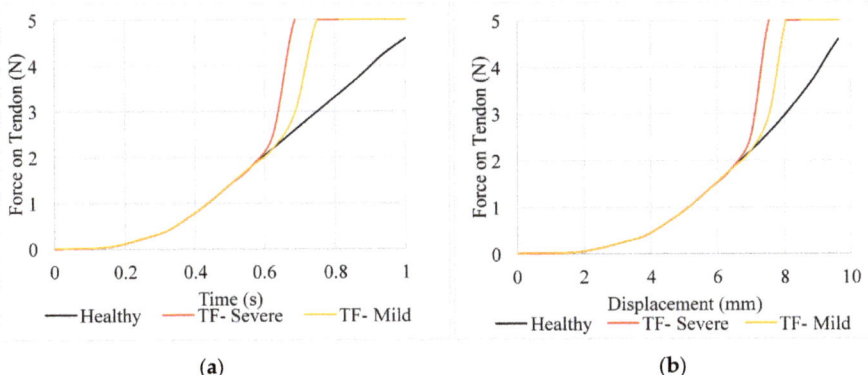

Figure 6. Force predicted for the FDP and FDS tendons (position B). (**a**) Force against time, (**b**) force against displacement.

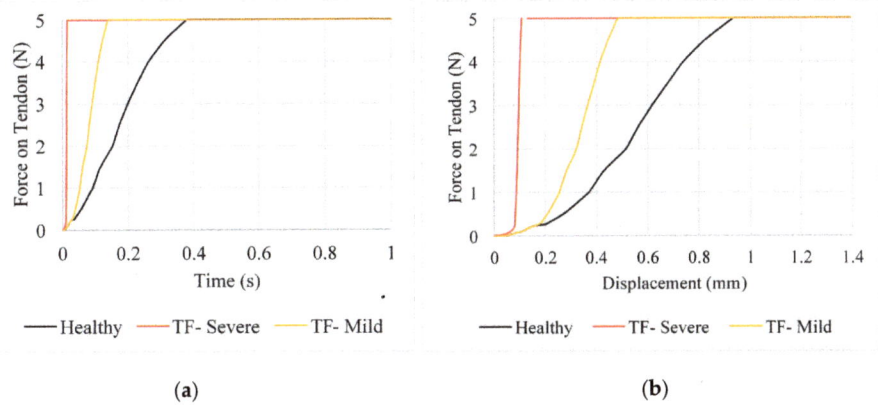

Figure 7. Force predicted for the FDP and FDS tendons (position C). (**a**) Force against time, (**b**) force against displacement.

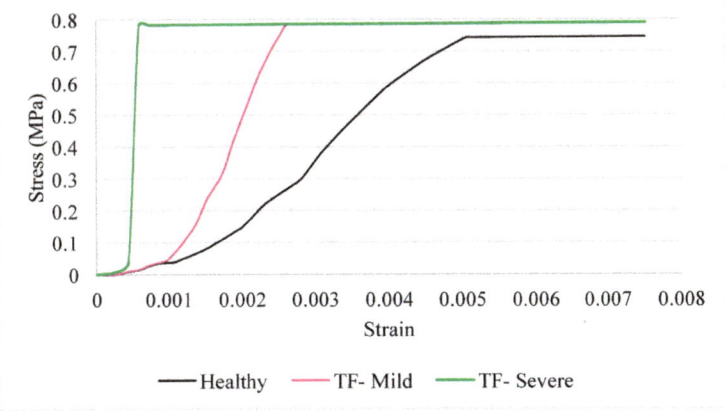

Figure 8. Stress–strain predicted for the FDP and FDS tendons (position C).

2.2. Position A—Extension

The locking of the tendon, caused by trigger finger, had a notable effect on the forces exerted in the tendons. In the case of severe trigger finger, a sharp increase in exerted force is observed at the point at which the tendon is restricted, in contrast to the healthy tendon where force increases gradually over time (Figures 2 and 3). There are much greater forces on the severely affected tendons as compared to those of the mildly affected tendon and the healthy tendon at the same displacement. For example, at 0.1 mm, forces are ≥5 N for the case of severe trigger finger, whereas, for the mildly affected and healthy tendon, the forces are 3.6 and 1.83 N, respectively. Healthy and affected tendons followed a linear stress–strain relationship until triggering, with a Young's modulus of approximately 1.5 MPa [24].

For the EDC tendon (Figure 4), the increase in force in the mildly affected tendon is less as compared to the equivalent condition for the FDS tendon (Figure 5). For example, a large increase in the measured force in the mildly affected tendon only noticeably increases at 0.38 mm for the EDC tendon, whereas, for the FDS tendon, the increase is immediate.

2.3. Position B—Abduction

Displacement of the tendons themselves was negligible during abduction for position B. For this motion, measuring the displacement of each node from its initial position provided much clearer results. Comparing the force–displacement graph for position B (Figure 6) to that of the extended finger in position A (Figure 3), the finger is able to undergo a larger displacement before an increase in force is observed. For the severe case of trigger finger in position B, force starts to increase rapidly at a displacement of 6.98 mm and at 7.53 mm for the mild trigger finger. Additionally, the rate of increase in force for severe trigger finger does not differ from that of the healthy tendon until 0.625 s, whereas the equivalent point was observed at 0.3125 s in position A.

2.4. Position C—Hyper-Extension

For position C, up to the point at which locking occurs in the severely affected tendon at 0.08 mm (Figure 7), measured force increases rapidly, similar to the force increase in position A (Figure 3). The change in force gradient was noticeably lower for the mildly affected tendon when approaching the 5 N limit, with an initial rise at 0.18 mm.

A "toe" region is observed in the stress–strain curves (Figure 8) of the hyper-extension movement of the finger before the relationship becomes linear. The mildly affected tendon can withstand a greater amount of strain over a longer period before triggering occurs. The mildly affected tendon reached a strain of 0.26% at the maximum stress of 0.78 MPa, whereas the severely affected tendon only reaches a strain of 0.059%.

2.5. Cross-Sectional Area and Tension

The cross-sectional area (CSA) of the tendons decreased when loads were applied (Table 1). As a result of the severely affected tendon's force increasing more rapidly before movement is restricted, the CSA is much greater than that of the mildly affected tendon, which has a much greater capacity to extend before finger movement is restrained. This is also the case for the tension in the tendons presented in Table 2. Tension in the mildly affected tendon in both positions was more than double that in the severely affected tendons, due to their greater capacity to extend.

Table 1. The calculated values for cross-sectional area, comparing positions A and C. Using Equations (1)–(7).

Tendon	Initial	Position A—Extension (mm²)			Position C—Hyper-Extension (mm²)		
		Healthy	Mild	Severe	Healthy	Mild	Severe
FDP	6.76	6.74	-	-	6.72	-	-
FDS	6.39	-	6.37	6.38	-	6.36	6.38
EDC	2.58	-	2.57	2.57	-	-	-

Table 2. The calculated values for tension, comparing positions A and C. Using Equations (1)–(7).

Tendon	Position A—Extension (N)			Position C—Hyper-Extension (N)		
	Healthy	Mild	Severe	Healthy	Mild	Severe
FDP	2.00	-	-	4.70	-	-
FDS	-	1.54	0.50	-	2.67	0.78
EDC	-	2.64	0.56	-	-	-

3. Discussion

This study has highlighted a clear increase in exerted force on tendons restricted by trigger finger when compared to healthy tendons under the same range of motion. The force analysis further indicates that the more severe the condition, the greater the stress induced in the tendon.

As expected, tension was higher when the tendons were under hyper-extension as compared to extension (position C vs. position A). Even for the healthy tendon, tension for position C (4.70 N) was measured to be more than double that at position A (2.00 N). This is in alignment with evidence found in the literature that demonstrates that hyper-extension injuries can occur when tendons or ligaments become overstretched [11]. In the case of trigger finger, greater tension was observed in the FDS tendon for position C as compared to position A (1.13 N greater under mild trigger finger). Further tendon injury could occur during hyper-extension as a result of trigger finger; tendons could become ruptured or separated from the bone, resulting in disrupted muscle function and joint instability.

For validation of the healthy tendon, several studies have been reviewed. Yang et al. [25] and Tanaka et al. [26] both tested this using tendons taken from fresh cadavers, whereas Kursa et al. [27] and Edsfeldt et al. [28] carried out testing during open carpal tunnel surgery. These studies all reported on loading forces during flexion. Loading forces on each joint in full flexion in the study by Yang et al. ranged from 1.69 to 7.93 N [25]. The forces in the study by Kursa et al. [27] ranged from 1.3 to 4 N in FDP tendons and 1.3–8.5 N in FDS tendons, and Edsfeldt et al. [28] reported forces of up to 13 N. Although the lock constraints may have meant that the model in our study has under-predicted the highest values for force, the results for the healthy FDP observed a trend which appears consistent with the maximum force values reported in the literature.

There are limitations to using cadaver models; for instance, specimens might be embalmed or treated with chemicals to prevent degradation, embalming may increase stiffness of the tissue [29,30], and treatments such as dehydration [31] and cross-linking (e.g., using glutaraldehyde) alter the physical and mechanical properties of tissues. If samples undergo freeze-thaw cycles, this too may alter their mechanical properties [32,33]. In the case of cross-linking, chemicals such as glutaraldehyde reduce degradation through the process of cross-linking of collagen, with a side-effect of increased stiffness, though this may depend on the state of crimp of the collagen which has undergone cross-linking [34].

When considering the forces acting on the FDS tendon during trigger finger, the results in this study were compared with Lu et al. [23]. The results from this study are particularly meaningful as it is the only study detailing the direct correlation between trigger finger and its effect on the forces acting on the tendon. External force increased gradually as extension angle increased; as triggering occurred, there was an abrupt increase in force, with the maximum force reaching 5.4 N. This coincides with results from this study, with peak values of around 5 N, which implies that any limitations in using connector elements may account for less than 10% of peak predictions. Therefore, this model is in agreement with the results found in the literature for extension.

One of the most common treatments for trigger finger is splinting; the affected finger is tied to a splint to restrict movement in flexion and extension while not restricting movement in abduction and adduction. For both the mildly and severely affected tendons, a displacement of 6.9 mm was reached before a sudden increase in observed force. These findings imply that there may be value in early treatment and the necessity of healthy tendons, providing further understanding of the impact of trigger finger to avoid the need for surgery. It is noteworthy that the current conservative treatment is splinting and physiotherapy; therefore, there is clear scope for innovation in this field. Active devices could be developed which enable the appropriate loading of tendons within the hand, potentially with a limit on loading/extension as necessary, e.g., to prevent hyper-extension, etc. One option for an active, external prosthetic device could be the use of electroactive polymers. There is also the possibility to combine this technology with micro-electro-mechanical systems to sense loading. Such a device could potentially be used at home, with data recorded and logged so that, during visits to the clinic, data could be evaluated—for instance, using a radio frequency identification (RFID) tag.

There is agreement in the literature that tension in the FDP tendon is greater than that in the FDS tendon for healthy fingers [25,27]. More specifically, in a study by Lu et al., tension generated during passive extension modelling was estimated in the FDP tendon as 1.41 to 22.93 N compared to 0.78 to 11.97 N in the FDS tendon [23]. If the FDS tendon is inflamed, as experimented with in this study, the overall strain on the FDP tendon would be greater, leading to significant long-term damage. Larger moments are necessary about the joints with trigger finger, so if there is an increase in repetitive high tendon loads, further deformation may occur. Tendons may also suffer elongation with sustained loads. There is less strain on both flexor tendons with mild trigger finger.

Ultimately, the intention of this paper is partly to encourage innovation for prosthetic devices to treat trigger finger, by providing a framework for initial stage development in silico. Patient specific models [35] can be useful to tailor any technologies to individuals. Alternatively, there is scope to scale the model used in this study to more quickly enable the clinical assessment of tension for a given individual; such scalable models have been of value in other areas of orthopaedics [36]. Setting up these types of models is feasible by producing scripts which generate input files directly and request input data such as boundary conditions in a specific format (e.g., .dat files) to then enable the FEA software to perform the numerical solution. Boundary conditions for models can also use boundary conditions specific to an individual [37]. One advantage of the generation of any computer-aided design model is that it can be 3D printed [38], which can also be useful for evaluation or interaction with patients when explaining the condition.

4. Materials and Methods

4.1. Geometry

A geometric model of a human skeleton was sourced [39] (Figure 9) and imported into computer-aided design software (SolidWorks, Dassault Systémes, Vélizy-Villacoublay, France), from which the hand bone structure was extracted. The bones were scaled using Solidworks; scaling was implemented so as to match the dimensions of an adult female available from the literature [40] (Table 3). The distal, middle and proximal phalanges and the metacarpal bone of the index finger were saved as separated parts before being imported into ABAQUS (Dassault Systems, Providence, RI, USA) as three-dimensional (3D) deformable components. The tendons and ligaments were then modelled using connector elements and constraints.

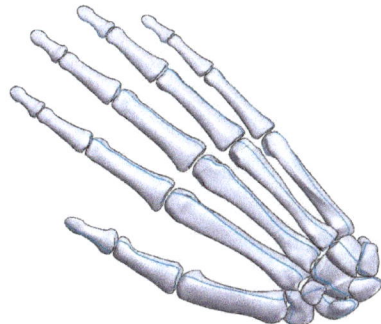

Figure 9. CAD model of the right hand used for simulations.

Table 3. The phalangeal and metacarpal lengths used in the CAD model.

Length (mm)			
Distal	Middle	Proximal	Metacarpal
24.1	34.5	56.1	104.7

4.2. Material Properties

The material properties for cortical bone [41] were assigned to each component, as detailed in Table 4. Ligaments and tendons are comprised of bundles of closely packed collagen fibrils [42–45], organised in parallel to resist strong tensile loads. Therefore, tendons, for instance, display hyperelastic properties, and as the finger is straightened in response to an applied load, the tendons start to deform in a linear fashion and become aligned [45].

Table 4. The properties of cortical bone implemented into the ABAQUS model; from the literature [41].

Property	Value
Young's Modulus	17 GPa
Poisson's Ratio	0.3
Density	1900 kg/m^3

Tendons were assumed to be incompressible, with no change in volume. Additionally, tendons were modelled as undergoing frictionless motion through the tendon sheath. However, where trigger finger was included in a simulation, the motion was restricted, as explained in Section 4.3.2. The path of the tendon was assumed to follow a straight line along the surface of the bone between two points in the tendon network. The loads experienced by a tendon were assumed to be distributed uniformly throughout the tendon network. Tendons were modelled using material properties from the literature [46]; this data was inputted directly into the ABAQUS, such as the data shown in Figure 10.

4.3. Model Set-Up

4.3.1. Joint Orientation

A kinematic model of the hand can be mathematically approximated as a number of revolute joints that are linked together. The index finger model is based on methods commonly used in the literature [1,47,48]. The distal (DIP) and proximal interphalangeal (PIP) joints have one degree-of-freedom (DOF) and are modelled as frictionless hinge joints capable of flexion-extension motion. The metacarpophalangeal (MCP) joint represents two DOF and is modelled as a frictionless saddle joint capable of flexion-extension and adduction-abduction. Coordinate systems were defined for each bone in the index finger with respect to a common inertial frame of reference to provide orientation of the joints and tendon configuration. A coordinate system for the distal, middle and proximal phalanx was used [49]. Each system is located in the centre of rotation in the convex articular surfaces of the phalangeal and metacarpal heads. The x-axis is projected along the shaft of the bones, with the y-axis projected dorsally and the z-axis projected radially for the right hand (note: these frames of reference are local to each individual bone).

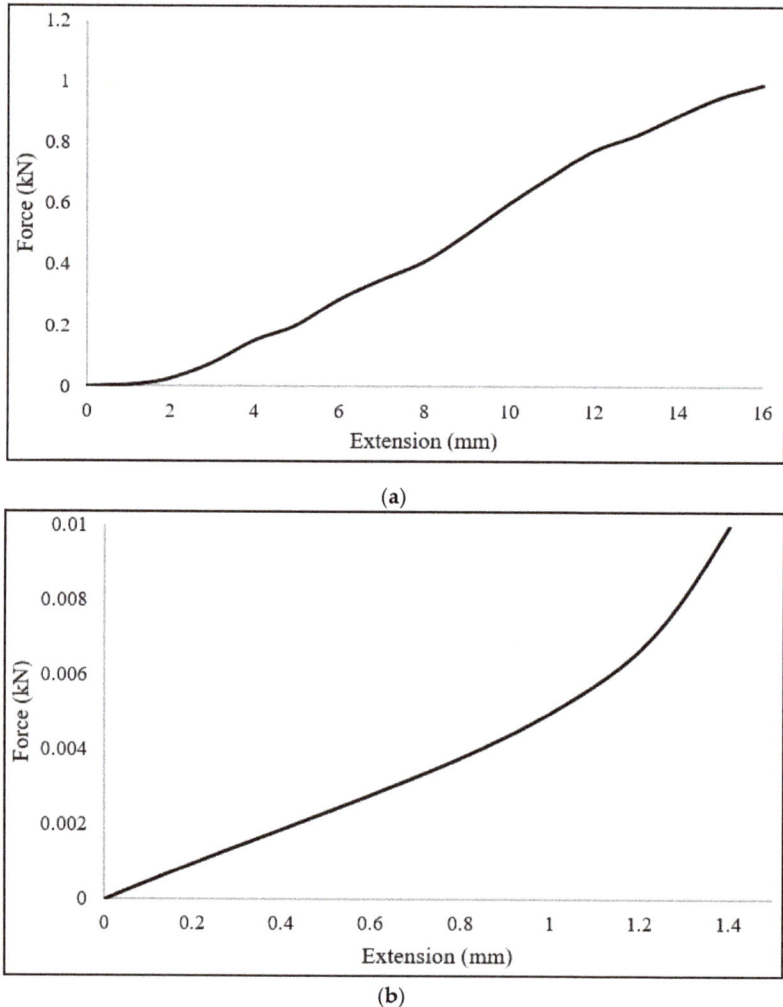

Figure 10. Sample force-extension data used to simulate tendons. (**a**) Full data set used from the literature [46]; (**b**) portion of the data relevant to the loading range within the simulations solved.

Initially, the phalanges were arranged in a flexed position [48] to resemble how the finger may be immobilised in the "trigger" position (Figure 11). Constraints were applied to ensure that each bone moved in the appropriate DOF and rotated accordingly within each coordinate system. A reference point was assigned at the centre of each convex surface of the bones. A coupling constraint was used which provides a coupling between a reference point and a group of nodes, with the necessary DOF applied between the articular surfaces. This ensures that the distal bone to the convex surface would only rotate about this surface. A general multi-point constraint (MPC) was used between each bone to ensure movement between bones was coordinated. The MPC was applied between the reference point and articular surface of each of the bones. This meant that only two displacement/rotation boundary conditions were necessary for the whole model, one to extend the finger and another to simultaneously straighten the distal phalanx.

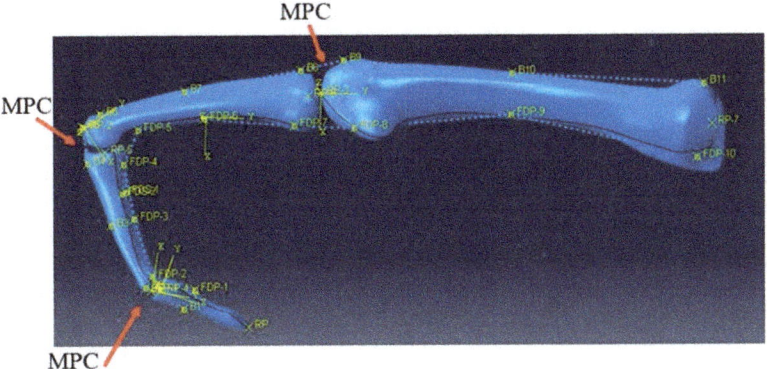

Figure 11. The initial flexed position of the index finger with the locations of multi-point constraints (MPCs) labelled.

4.3.2. Tendon and Ligament Modelling

Tendons and ligaments were simulated within the model as connector elements and constraints. Following the meshing of the bone structures, nodes were placed on the mesh at points of attachment in the tendons. To replicate the tendons being constricted by ligaments along the bone, connector elements were joined between the nodes on the bone. Nodes were spread evenly along the palmar and posterior aspects of the finger (Figure 12a).

Table 5. A table presenting the different movement-types investigated.

Position	Diagram	Description
Initial	Radial view	Flexed
A	Radial view	Extended from PIP joint (rotation about the z-axis)
B	Dorsal view	Extended before abduction from MCP joint (rotation about the y-axis)
C	Radial view	Extended then hyperextended from MCP joint (rotated further about the z-axis)

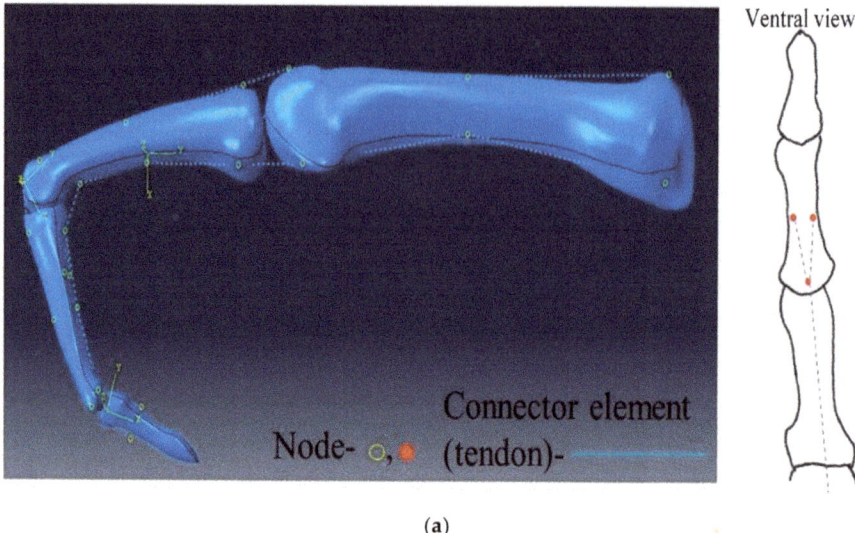

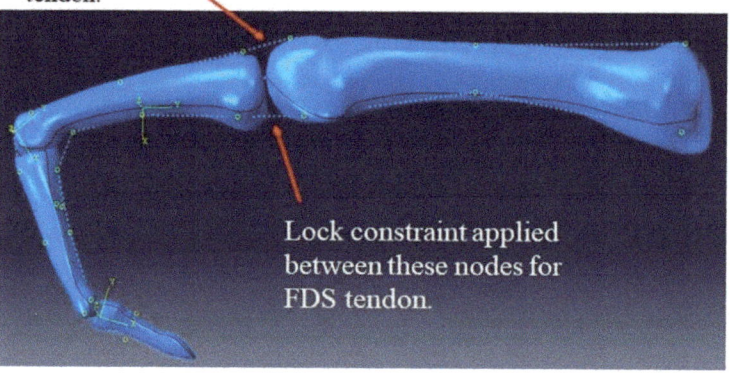

Figure 12. Connector elements used. (**a**) The positioning of the nodes and connector elements on the bones (the right image shows the nodes for the FDS tendon). (**b**) The locations of the lock constraints on the connector elements on the FDS and EDC tendons. Please refer to Table 5 for the movements mimicked.

Connector elements were placed so as to mimic the FDP tendon extending from the distal phalanx to the proximal end of the metacarpal, with the FDS tendon attaching to the middle phalanx in a forked arrangement. The FDS tendon is also constrained by the same set of nodes as the FDP tendon to the proximal metacarpal, both on the palm side. The FDP, FDS and EDC tendons were all modelled in the simulation, with the EDC tendon extending along the full length of the back of the finger, similarly held in place by nodes. A lock constraint as part of the connector element was applied on the FDS and

EDC tendons between the two nodes on either side of the MCP joint (Figure 12b). This is a common area in which tendons can experience irritation and consequently inflammation and restriction [50].

Lock constraints restrict movement after a set displacement; the displacement is the change in distance from one node to another. In this study, an estimate was made for the displacement of the lock based on the length of a flexor tendon in an index finger of an adult female. Displacement was set at 0.1 mm for severe trigger finger for relatively no movement and 0.5 mm for mild trigger finger to allow for some movement; 0.1 mm was used to avoid modelling artefacts which became evident when 0 mm was used in preliminary models, and 0.5 mm was used to determine how greater movement would alter tension and the timing of tension which would develop in tendons. To model a lock constraint in ABAQUS, two parameters are needed: firstly, a parameter being constrained (in this case, displacement at 0.1 or 0.5 mm) and a parameter which enforces this constraint (e.g., force). Preliminary models found that a 5 N load suitably enforced the lock constraint on displacement (of both 0.1 and 0.5 mm).

The movements evaluated are outlined in Table 5. For each movement type, results were taken for both severe and mild cases of trigger finger. Initially, the FDP and EDC tendons were modelled without any of the restrictions of trigger finger, whereas the FDS tendon became locked after the specified displacement. Starting from the initial flexed position, the finger was extended for position A, abducted for position B and hyperextended for position C.

4.3.3. Boundary Conditions

The movements outlined in Section 4.3.2 were feasible through the use of the boundary conditions outlined in Table 6. The metacarpal bone is stationary throughout the running of the simulation; therefore, an initial boundary condition of encastre was applied. In all positions, the finger started in the initial flexed position. For position A, the middle phalanx was rotated 96° about the z-axis until the finger was aligned to a straight orientation. The distal phalanx followed this direction of motion due to the MPC constraints and was simultaneously rotated 61° about the z-axis. The proximal phalanx was rotated 40° about the y-axis, simulating abduction for position B. After returning to the initial position, the finger was hyper-extended, rotating the proximal phalanx 45° about the z-axis.

Table 6. A list of the boundary conditions used in ABAQUS. U1, U2 and U3 specify movements along Table 1. UR2 and UR3 specify rotation about the x, y and z axes, respectively.

Boundary Condition	Step	Type	Bone(s)	Value (Rotation in Radians)
Position A				
Initial	Initial	Encastre	Metacarpal	U1, U2, U3 = 0
			Proximal phalanx	UR1, UR2, UR3 = 0
1	1	Displacement/rotation	Middle phalanx	UR3 = 1.68
2	1	Displacement/rotation	Distal phalanx	UR3 = 1.06
Position B				
Initial	Initial	Encastre	Metacarpal	U1, U2, U3 = 0
				UR1, UR2, UR3 = 0
1	1	Displacement/rotation	Middle phalanx	UR3 = 1.68
2	1	Displacement/rotation	Distal phalanx	UR3 = 1.06
3	2	Displacement/rotation	Proximal phalanx	UR2 = 0.7
Position C				
Initial	Initial	Encastre	Metacarpal	U1, U2, U3 = 0UR1, UR2, UR3 = 0
1	1	Displacement/rotation	Proximal phalanx	UR3 = 2.47
2	1	Displacement/rotation	Distal phalanx	UR3 = 1.06

4.4. Analysis

The cross-sectional area of a flexor tendon mid-section can range from 8.36 to 14.44 mm² [51,52] for an index finger. For this simplified model, the assumption made was that the FDP, FDS and EDC all have an initial average circular cross-sectional area, A, taken from the literature [53] (Table 7).

Table 7. The initial values used for initial cross-sectional area, initial length and Young's modulus used in Equations (1)–(7).

	A (mm²)	L0 (mm)	E (MPa)
FDP	6.76	185	1.5
FDS	6.38	149	1.5
EDC	2.58	180	1.5

Assuming homogenous material properties, uniform stiffness k for collagen can also be adopted along the tendon length [53]. For convenience, the mean slack length of the tendon will equal the mean initial tendon length L_0. Equations (1)–(3) have been adapted from Freij et al. [54], Equation (4) from Vigouroux et al. [22] and Equations (5)–(7) from Young et al. [53] to calculate the actual cross-sectional area a, true stress σ and stiffness after each position. Where λ is the stretch ratio, L is the actual length and F is force given in ABAQUS.

$$\lambda = \frac{L}{L_0}, \tag{1}$$

$$a = \frac{A}{\lambda}, \tag{2}$$

$$\sigma = \frac{F}{a}, \tag{3}$$

The tension, T, in the tendons can be estimated by relating force on the tendon to its elongation.
The tension, T, in the tendons can be estimated by relating force on the tendon to its elongation through displacement using a quadratic function (Equation (4)).

$$T = k(L - L_0)^2, \tag{4}$$

Stiffness k is estimated using Equation (5), where E is the Young's modulus of the tendon, which has previously been reported as being approximately 1.5 MPa [24], where ε is strain and ΔL is extension.

$$k = \frac{AE}{L_0}, \tag{5}$$

$$\varepsilon = \frac{\Delta L}{L_0}, \tag{6}$$

$$E = \frac{\sigma}{\varepsilon}, \tag{7}$$

Equations (1)–(7) were used to calculate tension in the tendon, stress and strain. The displacement and force of the connector element in the model, between the two nodes either side of the MCP joint, have been used when evaluating the equations during movements A, B and C (Table 6) for the healthy FDP tendon and the mildly and severely affected FDS tendon. Additionally, for movement A, analysis included the EDC healthy, mildly and severely affected tendons. Table 7 contains the initial values used for Equations (1)–(7).

4.5. Mesh and Solution

The analysis was performed using ABAQUS. A dynamic, explicit solution type was used with one to two steps. A time period of one second was applied for each step with boundary conditions using a tabular amplitude. The geometric complexity of the bones favoured the use of an automatic tetrahedral mesh, deemed acceptable as the bones were not expected to undergo large deformation. Mesh convergence consisted of increasing the node seed size in equal steps and identifying the size at which it did not alter predictions of tension in tendons. Mesh convergence occurred at a seed-size of 4.5, which resulted in a mesh with 5123 elements (solution time: ~14.2 min). It should be noted that only the bone structures are actually meshed and, given the loading involved, these undergo deformation which is negligible (in essence, acting as rigid bodies); this is why mesh convergence has occurred using a low number of elements.

5. Conclusions

This study demonstrates the effects that trigger finger has on the extensor mechanism, and it predicts tendon loads as caused by trigger finger as compared to a "healthy" control case. There appears to be a substantial increase in tension during hyper-extension during trigger finger. It is hoped that the model presented could be used as a framework to enable more advanced treatment methods to be developed than currently available (e.g., prosthetic devices for rehabilitation).

Author Contributions: Conceptualization, D.M.E. and C.G.B.; methodology, H.I.R. and D.M.E.; software, H.I.R.; validation, H.I.R.; formal analysis, H.I.R.; investigation, H.I.R. and D.M.E.; data curation, H.I.R.; writing—original draft preparation, H.I.R. and D.M.E.; writing—review and editing, D.M.E., H.I.R. and C.G.B.; supervision, D.M.E. All authors have read and agreed to the published version of the manuscript.

Funding: This research received no external funding.

Conflicts of Interest: The authors declare no conflict of interest.

References

1. Yun, Y.; Agarwal, P.; Deshpande, A.D. Accurate, robust, and real-time pose estimation of finger. *J. Dyn. Syst. Meas. Control* **2015**, *137*, 034505.
2. Hu, D.; Ren, L.; Howard, D.; Zong, C. Biomechanical analysis of force distribution in human finger extensor mechanisms. *BioMed. Res. Int.* **2014**, *2014*, 743460. [CrossRef] [PubMed]
3. Langer, D.; Maeir, A.; Michailevich, M.; Applebaum, Y.; Luria, S. Using the international classification of functioning to examine the impact of trigger finger. *Disabil. Rehabil.* **2016**, *38*, 2530–2537. [PubMed]
4. Langer, D.; Maeir, A.; Michailevich, M.; Luria, S. Evaluating hand function in clients with trigger finger. *Occup. Ther. Int.* **2017**, *2017*, 9539206. [CrossRef]
5. Lindner-Tons, S.; Ingell, K. An alternative splint design for trigger finger. *J. Hand Ther.* **1998**, *11*, 206–208. [CrossRef]
6. Sbernardori, M.C.; Bandiera, P. Histopathology of the A1 pulley in adult trigger fingers. *J. Hand Surg.* **2007**, *32*, 556–559.
7. Miyamoto, H.; Miura, T.; Isayama, H.; Masuzaki, R.; Koike, K.; Ohe, T. Stiffness of the first annular pulley in normal and trigger fingers. *J. Hand Surg.* **2011**, *36*, 1486–1491. [CrossRef]
8. Doughlas, H.C.L.; Chin, D.H.; Jones, N.F. Repetitive motion hand disorders. *J. Calif. Dent. Assoc.* **2002**, *30*, 149–160.
9. Makkouk, A.H.; Oetgen, M.E.; Swigart, C.R.; Dodds, S.D. Trigger finger: Etiology, evaluation, and treatment. *Curr. Rev. Musculoskel Med.* **2008**, *1*, 92–96.
10. Colbourn, J.; Heath, N.; Manary, S.; Pacifico, D. Effectiveness of splinting for the treatment of trigger finger. *J. Hand Ther.* **2008**, *21*, 336–343. [CrossRef]
11. Best, T.J. Post-traumatic stenosing flexor tenosynovitis. *Can. J. Plast. Surg.* **2003**, *11*, 143–144. [CrossRef] [PubMed]
12. The British Society for Surgery of the Hand. Trigger Finger/Thumb. Available online: https://www.bssh.ac.uk/patients/conditions/18/trigger_fingerthumb (accessed on 10 March 2019).
13. NHS Wales. Trigger Finger. Available online: https://www.nhsdirect.wales.nhs.uk/encyclopaedia/t/article/triggerfinger (accessed on 18 April 2019).
14. NHS. Trigger Finger. Available online: https://www.nhs.uk/conditions/trigger-finger/ (accessed on 5 April 2019).

15. Li, Z.M.; Zatsiorsky, V.M.; Latash, M.L. The effect of finger extensor mechanism on the flexor force during isometric tasks. *J. Biomech.* **2001**, *34*, 1097–1102. [CrossRef]
16. Wilkinson, D.D.; Weghe, M.V.; Matsuoka, Y. An extensor mechanism for an anatomical robotic hand. In Proceedings of the International Conference on Robotics & Automation, Taipei, Taiwan, 14–19 September 2003; Volume 1, p. 243.
17. Hirt, B.; Seyhan, H.; Wagner, M. *Hand and Wrist Anatomy and Biomechanics: A Comprehensive Guide*; Thieme Medical Publishers, Incorporated: New York, NY, USA, 2016.
18. Amis, A. The mechanical properties of finger flexor tendons and development of stronger tendon suturing techniques. In *Advances in the Biomechanics of the Hand and Wrist*; Schuind, F., Garcia-Elias, M., An, K.N., Eds.; Springer: Boston, MA, USA, 1994; p. 41.
19. Chen, P.; Lin, C.; Jou, I.M.; Chieh, H.F.; Su, F.C.; Kuo, L.C. One Digit Interruption: The altered force patterns during functionally cylindrical grasping tasks in patients with trigger digits. *PLoS ONE* **2013**, *8*, e83632. [CrossRef] [PubMed]
20. Tung, W.L.; Kuo, L.C.; Lai, K.Y.; Jou, I.M.; Sun, Y.N.; Su, F.C. Quantitative evidence of kinematics and functional differences in different graded trigger fingers. *Clin. Biomech.* **2010**, *25*, 535–540. [CrossRef] [PubMed]
21. Langer, D.; Luria, S.; Michailevich, M.; Maeir, A. Long-term functional outcome of trigger finger. *J. Disabil. Rehabil.* **2016**, *40*, 90–95.
22. Vigouroux, L.; Quaine, F.; Labarre-Vila, A.; Moutet, F. Estimation of finger muscle tendon tensions and pulley forces during specific sport-climbing grip techniques. *J. Biomech.* **2006**, *39*, 2583–2592. [CrossRef]
23. Lu, S.; Kuo, L.; Jou, I. Quantifying catch-and-release: The extensor tendon force needed to overcome the catching flexors in trigger fingers. *J. Orthop. Res.* **2013**, *31*, 1130–1135. [CrossRef]
24. Weber, J.F.; Agur, A.M.R.; Fattah, A.Y.; Gordon, K.D.; Oliver, M.L. Tensile mechanical properties of human forearm tendons. *J. Hand Surg. (Eur. Vol.)* **2015**, *40*, 711–719. [CrossRef]
25. Yang, T.; Lu, S.; Lin, W.; Zhao, K.; Zhao, C.; An, K.N.; Jou, I.M.; Lee, P.Y.; Kuo, L.C.; Su, F.C. Assessing finger joint biomechanics by applying equal force to flexor tendons in vitro using a novel simultaneous approach. *PLoS ONE* **2016**, *11*, e0160301.
26. Tanaka, T.; Amadio, P.C.; Zhao, C.; Zobits, M.E.; An, K.N. Flexor digitorum profundus tendon tension during finger manipulation. *J. Hand Ther.* **2005**, *18*, 330–338. [CrossRef]
27. Kursa, K.; Lattanza, L.; Diao, E.; Rempel, D. In vivo flexor tendon forces increase with finger and wrist flexion during active finger flexion and extension. *Orthop. Res.* **2006**, *24*, 763–769. [CrossRef] [PubMed]
28. Edsfeldt, S.; Rempel, D.; Kursa, K.; Diao, E.; Lattanza, L. In vivo flexor tendon forces generated during different rehabilitation exercises. *J. Hand Surg.* **2015**, *40*, 705–710. [CrossRef]
29. Barberio, C.G.; Chaudhry, T.; Power, D.M.; Tan, S.; Lawless, B.M.; Espino, D.M.; Wilton, J.C. Towards viscoelastic characterisation of the human ulnar nerve: An early assessment using embalmed cadavers. *Med. Eng. Phys.* **2019**, *64*, 15–22. [PubMed]
30. Barberio, C.; Chaudhry, T.; Power, D.; Lawless, B.M.; Espino, D.M.; Tan, S.; Wilton, J.C. The effect of shoulder abduction and medial epicondylectomy on ulnar nerve strain. *J. Musculoskelet Surg. Res.* **2019**, *3*, 134–140. [CrossRef]
31. Burton, H.E.; Williams, R.L.; Espino, D.M. Effects of freezing, fixation and dehydration on surface roughness properties of porcine left anterior descending coronary arteries. *Micron* **2017**, *101*, 78–86. [CrossRef] [PubMed]
32. Burton, H.E.; Freij, J.M.; Espino, D.M. Dynamic viscoelasticity and surface properties of porcine left anterior descending coronary arteries. *Cardiovasc. Eng. Technol.* **2017**, *8*, 41–56. [CrossRef]
33. Burton, H.E.; Cullinan, R.; Jiang, K.; Espino, D.M. Multiscale three-dimensional surface reconstruction and surface roughness of porcine left anterior descending coronary arteries. *R. Soc. Open Sci.* **2019**, *6*, 190915. [CrossRef]
34. Constable, M.; Burton, H.E.; Lawless, B.M.; Gramigna, V.; Buchan, K.G.; Espino, D.M. Effect of glutaraldehyde based cross-linking on the viscoelasticity of mitral valve basal chordae tendineae. *BioMed. Eng. Online* **2018**, *17*, 93.
35. Öhman, C.; Espino, D.M.; Heinmann, T.; Baleani, M.; Delingette, H.; Viceconti, M. Subject-specific knee joint model: Design of an experiment to validate a multi-body finite element model. *Vis. Comput.* **2011**, *27*, 153–159. [CrossRef]

36. Lavecchia, C.E.; Espino, D.M.; Moerman, K.M.; Tse, K.M.; Robinson, D.; Lee, P.V.S.; Shepherd, D.E.T. Lumbar model generator: A tool for the automated generation of a parametric scalable model of the lumbar spine. *J. R. Soc. Interface* **2018**, *15*, 20170829. [CrossRef]
37. Bahraseman, H.G.; Hassani, K.; Navidbakhsh, M.; Espino, D.M.; Sani, Z.A.; Fatouraee, N. Effect of exercise on blood flow through the aortic valve: A combined clinical and numerical study. *Comput. Methods Biomech. Biomed. Eng.* **2014**, *17*, 1821–1834. [CrossRef] [PubMed]
38. Jewkes, R.; Burton, H.E.; Espino, D.M. Towards additive manufacture of functional, spline-based morphometric models of healthy and diseased coronary arteries: In vitro proof-of-concept using a porcine template. *J. Funct. Biomater.* **2018**, *9*, 15. [CrossRef] [PubMed]
39. Sterling, S. Human Skeleton Used for a Parametric Gait Study. Available online: https://grabcad.com/library/human-skeleton-used-for-a-parametric-gait-study-1 (accessed on 10 November 2018).
40. Jasuja, O.P.; Singh, G. Estimation of stature from hand and phalange length. *J. indian Acad. Forensic Med.* **2004**, *26*, 100–106.
41. Pal, S. Mechanical properties of biological materials. In *Design of Artificial Human Joints & Organs*; Pal, S., Ed.; Springer: Boston, MA, USA, 2014; p. 23.
42. Hooley, C.J.; McCrum, N.G.; Cohen, R.E. The viscoelastic deformation of tendon. *J. Biomech.* **1980**, *13*, 521–528. [CrossRef]
43. Pradas, M.M.; Calleia, R.D. Nonlinear viscolelastic behaviour of the flexor tendon of the human hand. *J. Biomech.* **1990**, *23*, 773–781. [CrossRef]
44. Proske, U.; Morgan, D.L. Tendon stiffness: Methods of measurement and significance for the control of movement. A review. *J. Biomech.* **1987**, *20*, 75–82. [CrossRef]
45. Woo, S.L.; Johnson, G.A.; Smith, B.A. Mathematical modelling of ligaments and tendons. *J. Biomech. Eng.* **1993**, *115*, 468–473.
46. Pring, D.J.; Amis, A.A.; Coombs, R.R. The mechanical properties of human flexor tendons in relation to artificial tendons. *J. Hand Surg. Br. Eur. Vol.* **1985**, *10*, 331–336. [CrossRef]
47. Brook, N.; Mizrahi, J.; Shoham, M.; Daya, J. A biomechanical model of index finger dynamics. *Med. Eng. Phys.* **1995**, *17*, 54–63.
48. Fok, K.S.; Chou, S.M. Development of a finger biomechanical model and its considerations. *J. Biomech.* **2010**, *43*, 701–713. [CrossRef]
49. An, K.N.; Chao, E.Y.; Cooney, W.P.; Linscheid, R.L. Normative model of human hand for biomechanical analysis. *J. Biomech.* **1979**, *12*, 775–788. [CrossRef]
50. Williams, M.; Temperley, D.; Murali, R. Radiology of the hand. *Orthop. Trauma* **2019**, *33*, 45–52. [CrossRef]
51. Ward, S.R.; Loren, G.J.; Lundberg, S.; Lieber, R.L. High stiffness of human digital flexor tendons is suited for precise finger positional control. *Neurophysiol* **2006**, *96*, 2815–2818. [CrossRef]
52. Boyer, M.I.; Meunier, M.D.; Lescheid, J.; Burns, M.E.; Gelberman, R.H.; Silva, M.J. The influence of cross-sectional area on the tensile properties of flexor tendons. *J. Hand Surg.* **2001**, *26*, 828–832. [CrossRef] [PubMed]
53. Young, S.R.; Gardiner, B.; Mehdizadeh, A.; Rubenson, J.; Umberger, B.; Smith, D.W. Adaptive remodeling of achilles tendon: A multi-scale computational model. *PLoS Comput. Biol.* **2016**, *12*, e1005106. [CrossRef]
54. Freij, J.M.; Burton, H.E.; Espino, D.M. Objective uniaxial identification of transition points in non-linear materials: Sample application to porcine coronary arteries and the dependency of their pre- and post-transitional moduli with position. *Cardiovasc. Eng. Technol.* **2019**, *10*, 61–68. [CrossRef]

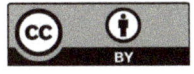 © 2020 by the authors. Licensee MDPI, Basel, Switzerland. This article is an open access article distributed under the terms and conditions of the Creative Commons Attribution (CC BY) license (http://creativecommons.org/licenses/by/4.0/).

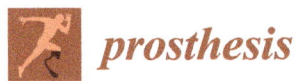

Editorial

Worldwide 3D Printers against the New Coronavirus

Luca Fiorillo [1,*] and Teresa Leanza [2]

1. Department of Biomedical and Dental Sciences, Morphological and Functional Images, University of Messina, Policlinico G. Martino, Via Consolare Valeria, 98100 Messina, Italy
2. Multidisciplinary Department of Medical-Surgical and Odontostomatological Specialties, University of Campania "Luigi Vanvitelli", 80100 Naples, Italy; teresa.leanza@policliniconapoli.it
* Correspondence: lfiorillo@unime.it

Received: 30 May 2020; Accepted: 4 June 2020; Published: 5 June 2020

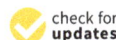

Abstract: The pandemic caused by the new coronavirus has placed national health systems of different countries in difficulty, and has demonstrated the need for many types of personal protective equipment (PPE). Thanks to the advent of new three-dimensional printing technologies, it was possible to share print files (using stereolithography (stl)) quickly and easily, improve them cooperatively, and allow anyone who possessed the materials, a suitable 3D printer and these files, to print. The possibility of being able to print three-dimensional supports, or complete personal protective equipment has been of incredible help in the management of COVID-19 (Coronavirus Disease 2019). The times and the relatively low costs have allowed a wide diffusion of these devices, especially for the structures that needed them, mainly healthcare facilities. 3D printing, now includes different fields of application, and represents, thanks to the evolution of methods and printers, an important step towards the "digital world".

Keywords: coronavirus; COVID-19; 3D-printing; DPI; protection; public health

---

Three-dimensional printers and millers are now widely used in the world; both in the medical field and in other areas such as electronics, engineering, construction, and military fields [1]. Technological development has made it possible to print (or mill) different materials, with multiple characteristics, and with good resolutions and reliability compared to analogue techniques [2–4]. 3D (3 dimensional) printing (or additive manufacturing) allows the creation, starting from a digital model, of three-dimensional physical objects, by depositing, layer by layer, of overlying materials. 3D printing dates back to the 80s. Beginnings could be considered with stereolithography (rapid prototyping and STL (STereo Lithography) format), followed by sintering (selective laser sintering), to arrive at fused deposition modeling or 3D printing with molten material [5,6]; it was thanks to the three dimensional printing that it became possible to print in color, while with the Electron beam melting, or even electron beam fusion, it was possible to obtain metal objects with a high density [7,8].

At the end of 2019, scientists isolated a new coronavirus in these subjects, designated SARS-CoV-2 (Severe Acute Respiratory Syndrome—Coronavirus-2), found to be similar to at least 70% of its gene sequence to that of SARS-CoV. Patients experience flu-like symptoms such as fever, dry cough, tiredness, difficulty breathing [9–15]. Certainly, the most common methods of diffusion of the virus involve the spread of infected droplets at a distance, through coughing, sneezing, or simply speaking. In more severe cases, often found in subjects already burdened by previous pathologies, pneumonia develops, acute renal failure, up to even death. 3D printing has found wide application in the medical field also in the Covid-19 (Coronavirus Disease—2019) emergency period. In fact, given the difficulty in finding official health supplies, thanks to this technology, many people have mobilized in a completely autonomous way to find concrete solutions. The whole world of "markers" and digital companies has exploited 3D printers in order to make up for these shortcomings by creating spare parts, fittings and compatible tubes for medical instruments in record time, useful for dealing with emergencies [16–19]. Recently, doctors, running out of valves for respiratory intensive care equipment and unable to purchase them from companies, needed to find a solution to save the lives of hospitalized patients.

This impactful event shone the spotlight on the activity within the community made up of makers and producers, which for some time had started to make a contribution to the health emergency, starting to organize itself to produce materials missing or that it would have been better to manufacture on site to avoid delivery delays. In fact, to print in 3D it is not enough to connect a machine to the internet. However, you also need:

- The printing material, which can be powder or filament of plastic, metal, ceramic or other;
- The so-called post-production, or someone who takes care of pulling the piece out of the machine, eliminating the supports, the unnecessary parts, cleaning it from extra dust and, if necessary, finishing it.

In a short time, makers and big producers came to organize themselves to have everything quickly. CAD (Computer Aided Design) files of all types have sprung up at the makers' sites, from valves to face masks. On Facebook® the communities and groups in which people recommend the best materials, the most effective design and so on have multiplied too. University researchers are contributing to efforts in various centers of excellence. Finally, companies that supply pieces to complement those printed, such as fabrics or screens for protective masks, have accelerated their production and donated materials to the Italian regions (as Decathlon® did with its snorkeling masks). In short, the market has been populated with alternatives and solutions, giving life to an extraordinary offer, albeit very varied in terms of quality [20–26].

Especially when it comes to medical devices and personal protective equipment, European consumer protection legislation is very strict and requires a long process of certification before being placed on the market. For example, some protective equipment may require approval by the Food and Drug Administration (FDA). Therefore, it must be ensured that companies that deal with additive manufacturing have a pass to continue their activity even during the lockdown period. At the international level, the flow of data (and therefore the design of 3D printed objects) should continue to be free of localization policies, barriers and duties. 3D printing has undoubted advantages when it comes to small productions, custom objects or complex designs. The additive manufacturing cancels the adaptation and configuration times of the machines (such as those for the creation of new molds), and allows the creation of complex and customized pieces without splitting up costs and production times [27]. It therefore remains to be understood how, once the emergency has passed, people may be able to take advantage of the specific benefits of this technology and whether its use in crisis situations will push for a more widespread adoption.

Author Contributions: Validation, T.L., project administration, L.F. All authors have read and agreed to the published version of the manuscript.

Funding: This research received no external funding.

Acknowledgments: In this COVID-19 emergency period, thanks go to all clinicians and researchers who everyday risk their lives for research.

Conflicts of Interest: The authors declare no conflict of interest.

References

1. Hodson, R. Digital revolution. *Nature* **2018**, *563*, S131. [CrossRef] [PubMed]
2. Cervino, G.; Fiorillo, L.; Arzukanyan, A.V.; Spagnuolo, G.; Cicciu, M. Dental Restorative Digital Workflow: Digital Smile Design from Aesthetic to Function. *Dent. J.* **2019**, *7*, 30. [CrossRef] [PubMed]
3. Lavorgna, L.; Cervino, G.; Fiorillo, L.; Di Leo, G.; Troiano, G.; Ortensi, M.; Galantucci, L.; Cicciù, M. Reliability of a virtual prosthodontic project realized through a 2d and 3d photographic acquisition: An experimental study on the accuracy of different digital systems. *Int. J. Environ. Res. Public Health* **2019**, *16*, 5139. [CrossRef] [PubMed]

4. Cicciù, M.; Fiorillo, L.; D'Amico, C.; Gambino, D.; Amantia, E.M.; Laino, L.; Crimi, S.; Campagna, P.; Bianchi, A.; Herford, A.S.; et al. 3D Digital Impression Systems Compared with Traditional Techniques in Dentistry: A Recent Data Systematic Review. *Materials* **2020**, *13*, 1982. [CrossRef] [PubMed]
5. American Association for the Advancement of Science. Playing With Epidemics. *Science* **2007**, *316*, 961. [CrossRef]
6. Cervino, G.; Montanari, M.; Santonocito, D.; Nicita, F.; Baldari, R.; De Angelis, C.; Storni, G.; Fiorillo, L. Comparison of Two Low-Profile Prosthetic Retention System Interfaces: Preliminary Data of an In Vitro Study. *Prosthesis* **2019**, *1*, 54–60. [CrossRef]
7. Han, X.; Yang, D.; Yang, C.; Spintzyk, S.; Scheideler, L.; Li, P.; Li, D.; Geis-Gerstorfer, J.; Rupp, F. Carbon Fiber Reinforced PEEK Composites Based on 3D-Printing Technology for Orthopedic and Dental Applications. *J. Clin. Med.* **2019**, *8*, 240. [CrossRef]
8. Pizzicannella, J.; Diomede, F.; Gugliandolo, A.; Chiricosta, L.; Bramanti, P.; Merciaro, I.; Orsini, T.; Mazzon, E.; Trubiani, O. 3D Printing PLA/Gingival Stem Cells/ EVs Upregulate miR-2861 and -210 during Osteoangiogenesis Commitment. *Int. J. Mol. Sci.* **2019**, *20*, 3256. [CrossRef]
9. Kobayashi, T.; Jung, S.-M.; Linton, N.M.; Kinoshita, R.; Hayashi, K.; Miyama, T.; Anzai, A.; Yang, Y.; Yuan, B.; Akhmetzhanov, A.R.; et al. Communicating the Risk of Death from Novel Coronavirus Disease (COVID-19). *J. Clin. Med.* **2020**, *9*, 580. [CrossRef]
10. Veltkamp, H.-W.; Akegawa Monteiro, F.; Sanders, R.; Wiegerink, R.; Lötters, J. Disposable DNA Amplification Chips with Integrated Low-Cost Heaters †. *Micromachines* **2020**, *11*, 238. [CrossRef]
11. Wang, C.; Pan, R.; Wan, X.; Tan, Y.; Xu, L.; Ho, C.S.; Ho, R.C. Immediate Psychological Responses and Associated Factors during the Initial Stage of the 2019 Coronavirus Disease (COVID-19) Epidemic among the General Population in China. *Int. J. Environ. Res. Public Health* **2020**, *17*, 1729. [CrossRef] [PubMed]
12. Linton, N.M.; Kobayashi, T.; Yang, Y.; Hayashi, K.; Akhmetzhanov, A.R.; Jung, S.-M.; Yuan, B.; Kinoshita, R.; Nishiura, H. Incubation Period and Other Epidemiological Characteristics of 2019 Novel Coronavirus Infections with Right Truncation: A Statistical Analysis of Publicly Available Case Data. *J. Clin. Med.* **2020**, *9*, 538. [CrossRef] [PubMed]
13. Ashour, H.M.; Elkhatib, W.F.; Rahman, M.M.; Elshabrawy, H.A. Insights into the Recent 2019 Novel Coronavirus (SARS-CoV-2) in Light of Past Human Coronavirus Outbreaks. *Pathogens* **2020**, *9*, 186. [CrossRef] [PubMed]
14. Allam, Z.; Jones, D.S. On the Coronavirus (COVID-19) Outbreak and the Smart City Network: Universal Data Sharing Standards Coupled with Artificial Intelligence (AI) to Benefit Urban Health Monitoring and Management. *Healthcare* **2020**, *8*, 46. [CrossRef]
15. Crimi, S.; Fiorillo, L.; Bianchi, A.; D'Amico, C.; Amoroso, G.; Gorassini, F.; Mastroieni, R.; Marino, S.; Scoglio, C.; Catalano, F.; et al. Herpes Virus, Oral Clinical Signs and QoL: Systematic Review of Recent Data. *Viruses* **2019**, *11*, 463. [CrossRef]
16. Fiorillo, L.; D'Amico, C.; Turkina, A.Y.; Nicita, F.; Amoroso, G.; Risitano, G. Endo and Exoskeleton: New Technologies on Composite Materials. *Prosthesis* **2020**, *2*, 1–9. [CrossRef]
17. Ortensi, L.; Vitali, T.; Bonfiglioli, R.; Grande, F. New Tricks in the Preparation Design for Prosthetic Ceramic Laminate Veneers. *Prosthesis* **2019**, *1*, 29–40. [CrossRef]
18. Cicciù, M. Prosthesis: New Technological Opportunities and Innovative Biomedical Devices. *Prosthesis* **2019**, *1*, 1–2. [CrossRef]
19. Cavallo, L.; Marcianò, A.; Cicciù, M.; Oteri, G. 3D Printing beyond Dentistry during COVID 19 Epidemic: A Technical Note for Producing Connectors to Breathing Devices. *Prosthesis* **2020**, *2*, 46–52. [CrossRef]
20. Calisher, C.; Carroll, D.; Colwell, R.; Corley, R.B.; Daszak, P.; Drosten, C.; Enjuanes, L.; Farrar, J.; Field, H.; Golding, J.; et al. Statement in support of the scientists, ublic health professionals, and medical professionals of China combatting COVID-19. *Lancet* **2020**. [CrossRef]
21. Spina, S.; Marrazzo, F.; Migliari, M.; Stucchi, R.; Sforza, A.; Fumagalli, R. The response of Milan's Emergency Medical System to the COVID-19 outbreak in Italy. *Lancet* **2020**, *395*, e49–e50. [CrossRef]
22. The, L. COVID-19: Fighting panic with information. *Lancet* **2020**, *395*, 537. [CrossRef]
23. Dong, E.; Du, H.; Gardner, L. An interactive web-based dashboard to track COVID-19 in real time. *Lancet Infect. Dis.* **2020**. [CrossRef]
24. Xu, B.; Kraemer, M.U.G. Open access epidemiological data from the COVID-19 outbreak. *Lancet Infect. Dis.* **2020**. [CrossRef]

25. Fiorillo, L.; Cervino, G.; De Stefano, R.; Iannello, G.; Cicciù, M. Socio-economic behaviours on dental profession: An in Italy google trends investigation. *Minerva Stomatol.* **2020**. [CrossRef]
26. Militi, A.; Cicciu, M.; Sambataro, S.; Bocchieri, S.; Cervino, G.; De Stefano, R.; Fiorillo, L. Dental occlusion and sport performance. *Minerva Stomatol.* **2020**. [CrossRef] [PubMed]
27. Makin, S. Searching for digital technology's effects on well-being. *Nature* **2018**, *563*, S138–S140. [CrossRef]

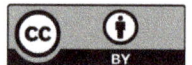 © 2020 by the authors. Licensee MDPI, Basel, Switzerland. This article is an open access article distributed under the terms and conditions of the Creative Commons Attribution (CC BY) license (http://creativecommons.org/licenses/by/4.0/).

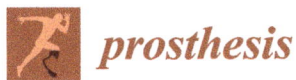

Article

3D Printing beyond Dentistry during COVID 19 Epidemic: A Technical Note for Producing Connectors to Breathing Devices

Leonardo Cavallo [1], Antonia Marcianò [2], Marco Cicciù [3,*] and Giacomo Oteri [3]

1. Master Dental Technician, Private Practice, 98050 Terme Vigliatore(ME), Italy; cavaleo72@gmail.com
2. Department of Clinical and Experimental Medicine, University of Messina, 98100 Messina, Italy; antmarciano@unime.it
3. Department of Biomedical and Dental Sciences and Morphofunctional Imaging, University of Messina, 98100 Messina, Italy; giacomo.oteri@unime.it
* Correspondence: acromarco@yahoo.it or mcicciu@unime.it

Received: 30 March 2020; Accepted: 3 April 2020; Published: 7 April 2020

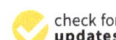

Abstract: (1) Background: To mitigate the shortage of respiratory devices during the Covid-19 epidemic, dental professional volunteers can contribute to create printed plastic valves, adapting the dental digital workflow and converting snorkeling masks in emergency CPAP (continuous positive airways pressure) devices. The objective of this report was to provide the specific settings to optimize printing with the 3D printers of the dental industry. (2) Methods: In order to provide comprehensive technical notes to volunteer dental professionals interested in printing Charlotte and Dave connectors to breathing devices, the entire digital workflow is reported. (3) Results: The present paper introduces an alternative use of the dental Computer Aided Design/Computer Aided Manufacturing (CAD/CAM) machinery, and reports on the fabrication of a 3D printed connection prototypes suitable for connection to face masks, thereby demonstrating the feasibility of this application. (4) Conclusions: This call for action was addressed to dentists and dental laboratories who are willing to making available their experience, facilities and machinery for the benefit of patients, even way beyond dentistry.

Keywords: Covid-19; CAD/CAM; 3D printing; dental prostheses; resin printed device

---

1. Introduction

The pandemic outbreak of a severe acute respiratory syndrome (SARS) associated with the novel coronavirus (2019-nCoV) poses a serious public health risk due to the high number of patients demand for ICU admission and mechanical ventilation [1,2].

To date (28 March 2020) in Italy 26,676 patients are hospitalized without mechanical ventilation, and 39,533 are advised to recover at home without continuous medical care, although in many of these cases, a support for spontaneous ventilation is needed [3].

CPAP (continuous positive airways pressure) allows the insufflation of air and oxygen at positive pressure in a continuous and non-invasive way for the duration of the respiratory cycle. The CPAP can be delivered through a mask (facial or nasal), flow and oxygen dispenser or with a mechanical fan. The choice of device depends on the patient's clinical condition, the environment in which it is delivered and the technological resources available [4].

In emergency settings, CPAP is an important alternative to invasive mechanical ventilation. Nevertheless, it can be used in several acute and chronic respiratory diseases, and also at home with a portable oxygen source, as provided in obstructive sleep apnea treatment [5].

At the moment, given the serious coronavirus pandemic, the majority of Italian hospitals do not have sufficient equipment to assist patients affected by respiratory failure, by reducing alveolar compression and supporting breathing [6].

In order to find an urgent solution to the need of respiratory devices, an Italian engineer (Dr. Eng. C. Fracassi) has ideated a respiratory device consisting of a commercially available snorkeling face mask *Easybreath* (Decathlon-Villeneuve-d'Ascq, France) in which the respiratory tube is replaced with a plastic support suitable to be connected to medical oxygen supply pipes.

The project of the connector has been designed by the Italian company ISINNOVA (Brescia, Italy), which has released on the web the related "standard triangulation language" STL files for free.

Consequently, in order to have the facial mask available for the conversion into a CPAP, it is necessary to apply the specifically designed fitting component consisting of two connection pieces that are printable with modern three-dimensional printers (3D).

The developed respiratory device is the result of the application of two 3D printed plastic valves *"Charlotte"* and *"Dave"* to the *Easybreath mask* (Model *Subea 1*).

The entire system set-up is made up as follows:

- Oxygen source
- Venturi valve
- *Dave* valve (to be connected with both inspiratory tube and reservoir)
- Connector tube
- *Charlotte* valve (to be connected to the inspiratory and expiratory branches of the breathing circuit)
- *Face mask* (in this case a snorkeling mask in which the internal valves direction needs to be reversed, allowing oxygen to flow inside) [7].
- Filter
- PEEP (positive end-expiratory pressure) valve

Considering the growing Covid-19 epidemic and the consequent exceptional case of necessity, the Italian Ministry of Health allows the use of these non-certified biomedical devices for compassionate care.

The application of an information procedure and a specific patient's informed consent is requested before using these devices [8].

Because of Covid-19, hospitals are urgently requesting breathing devices; groups of volunteers working in research centers, companies, individuals and among them also dentists and dental technicians have joined together to quickly create 3D printing fittings.

The present paper introduces an alternative use of the dental CAD/CAM machinery, reporting on the fabrication of a 3D printed connections prototype suitable for connection to snorkeling face masks, demonstrating the feasibility of the application. 3D printing companies act as central hubs connecting makers and hospitals in need by crowdsourcing a list of professional additive manufacturing (AM) providers who have suiTable 3D printers. Dentists and dental laboratories who are willing to making available their experience, facilities and machinery for the fight against the coronavirus can sign up at https://www.3dsystems.com/covid-19-response#signUp [9].

The objective of this report was to present the specific workflow to be applied for printing the connectors with Dental 3D Printers that meet the reported setting requirements. Medical-grade materials must be used.

2. Results

In order to provide comprehensive technical notes to volunteer dental professionals interested in printing Charlotte and Dave connectors to breathing devices, the entire digital workflow is reported.

Step by Step Procedure

The steps leading to the resulting pieces are described below.

The STL file available by ISINNOVA srl. of the *"Charlotte"* valve and *"Dave"* valve is imported to the 3D printer software(PreForm 3.4.3 Formlabs Inc.) (Figures 1 and 2).

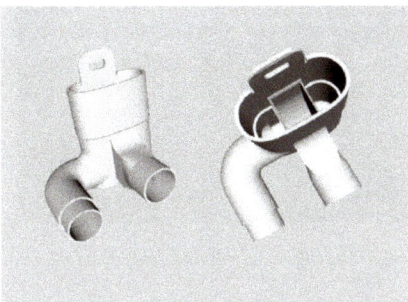

Figure 1. STL file of *"Charlotte"* valve (made available by ISINNOVA srl.).

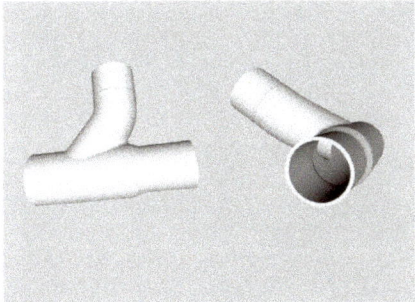

Figure 2. STL file of *"Dave"* valve (made available by ISINNOVA srl.).

The corrected position of the pieces in the printer plate (Figure 3) and the number, position, height and diameter of the supporting pins are checked according to instructions.

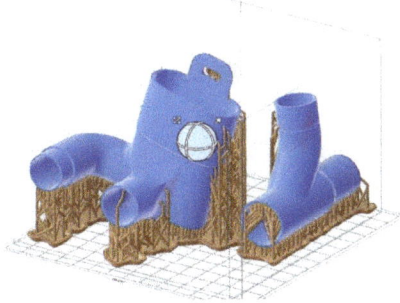

Figure 3. *"Charlotte"* and *"Dave"* valves leaning on the printer terminal plate.

The print is then launched at a predetermined operating time (5 h 15 min).

At the end of the printing, (Figure 4) a post-production phase is required.

The polymerized components are removed from the printer and washed in **Isopropyl alcohol** in an ultrasound tank for 5–15 min.

Subsequently, they are cured and dried in the UV curing system Meccatronicore BB Cure Dental (Meccatronicore, Trento, Italy).

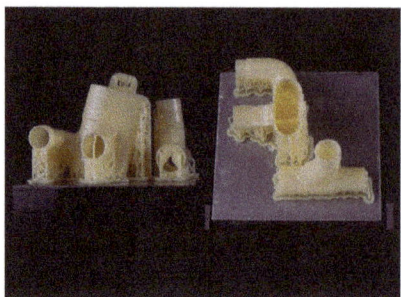

Figure 4. Printed vales external and internal vision.

All supporting pins are removed, and the external surfaces of the plastic devices are finished using conventional dental methods, with rotating burs and brushes (Figure 5).

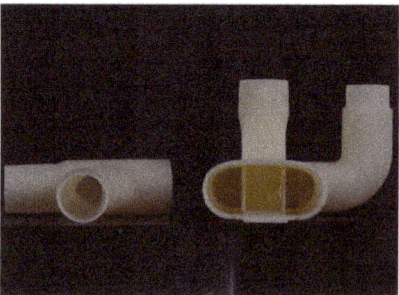

Figure 5. Finishing.

The last step is cleaning with a broad-spectrum disinfectant hydroalcoholic solution (**Bactisan Spray, Amedics**).

Finally, the valves, stored in sterilization tubing to avoid contamination, are ready for delivery, since correct adaptation to the mask is ensured. (Figures 6–8).

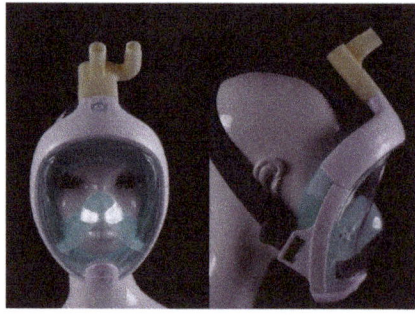

Figure 6. Insertion of "*Charlotte*" valve to the mask.

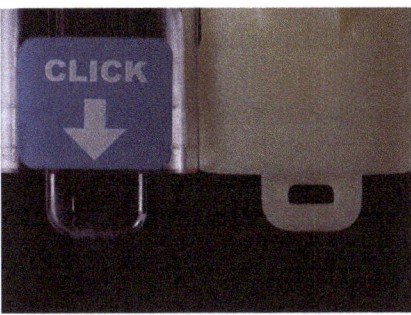

Figure 7. Printed connector detail comparison to *Subea 1*.

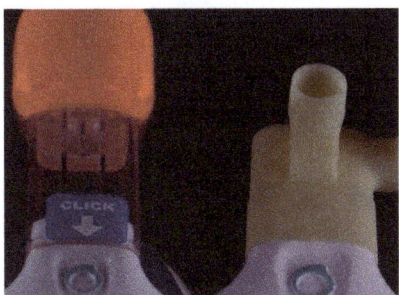

Figure 8. Comparison between *"Charlotte"* and *Subea* 1 insertion.

3. Discussion

The severe and widespread Covid-19 pandemic puts many people's lives at risk all over the world.

The insufficient number of beds in Intensive Care Units associated with the huge demand for assisted breathing devices cannot be met by factory supplies in a short time.

Alternative and emergency respiratory apparatuses can help the breathing of many patients who are affected by coronavirus.

However, it is noteworthy to mention that in Covid-19 patients with acute respiratory failure, CPAP may not be an adequate treatment. Therefore, since it is difficult to predict what these cases are, the decision to try this treatment is up to the intensive care specialist and they need to provide close monitoring, including preparations for prompt intubation.

3D printing translates computer-aided design (CAD) virtual 3D models into physical objects. 3D printing is used in the manufacturing industry, medical and pharmaceutical research, drug production, clinical medicine and dentistry, with implications for precision and personalized medicine [10,11].

The term 3D printing with the alias Customized Additive Manufacturing (AM) is used to describe the same general manufacturing principle that builds objects layer by layer.

AM techniques include vat photopolymerization (stereolithography), powder bed fusion (SLS), material and binder jetting (inkjet and aerosol 3D printing), sheet lamination (LOM), extrusion (FDM, 3D dispensing, 3D fiber deposition and 3D plotting) and 3D bio printing [12].

With the advent of computer-aided design/computer-aided manufacturing (CAD/CAM) protocols, it became quite popular in dentistry, especially for implant prosthodontics [13,14].

Dental professionals have a deep awareness of digital workflow for 3D printing, since the use of it to build dental models, fixed prostheses, full-arch implant supported rehabilitation and others is nowadays routine in the daily dental practice.

Volunteer dental professionals can contribute to creating printed plastic valves, adapting the dental digital workflow and converting snorkeling masks in emergency CPAP devices.

The role of the dentist and the dental laboratory is only limited to making available their experience, facilities and machinery for helping doctors and patients, even way beyond dentistry [15–17].

4. Materials and Methods

The free STL files of Charlotte and Dave valves were downloaded from the link: https://drive.google.com/drive/folders/14Q3TEl5JVeN2QpDpKo1AIx_wnGeolKlK?usp=sharing.

The low force stereolithography (LFS) Formlabs Form 2 printer (Formlabs Inc., Somerville, MA, USA) was used. Stereolithography is an additive manufacturing process that, in its most common form, works by focusing an ultraviolet (UV) laser on to a vat of photopolymer resin; the resin is photochemically solidified and forms a single layer of the desired 3D object from the computer-aided design (CAM/CAD) software. This process is repeated for each layer of the design until the 3D object is complete [13].

In the design phase, the option "automatically generates everything" allows us to take advantage of the pre-defined settings for the creation of the supports.

The following basic settings were used:

Density: 1.00
Size of the contact points: 0.90
Internal supports: on
Spacing from the plane: 5.00
Inclination multiplier: 1.00
Height above the base: 5.00
Base thickness: 2.00
Layer thickness: 0.1 mm
Print time: 5 h 15 min
Layers: 932
Volume: 60.52 mL

The printer is used in "open mod" activity to allow the use of resins other than the original ones supplied by Formlabs.

In this case, the employed printing material was NextDentTM C&B (NextDent B.V., 3769 AV Soesterberg, Netherlands), a micro filled hybrid (MFH) class II a printing material suitable for medical devices, biocompatible and CE certified in accordance with Medical Device Directive 93/42/EEC, listed by the FDA and registered in various other countries.

For this prototype, the color A 3,5 was chosen.

This material reflects the characteristics of the ideal material for this use, which should be odorless, biocompatible, biocomposable and relatively flexible to easily connect with the mask component.

Author Contributions: L.C. and A.M. equally conceived and designed the article; L.C. carried out the devices. G.O. drafted the manuscript and coordinated the study; M.C. critically revised the manuscript. All authors have read and agreed to the published version of the manuscript.

Funding: This research received no external funding.

Acknowledgments: Declare none.

Conflicts of Interest: The authors declare no conflict of interest.

References

1. COVID-19. Available online: https://www.ecdc.europa.eu/en/novel-coronavirus-china (accessed on 1 March 2020).

2. Outbreak of Novelcoronavirus Disease 2019(COVID-19): Situation in Italy. Available online: https://www.ecdc.europa.eu/sites/default/files/documents/novel-coronavirus-threat-assessment-brief-23-feb-2020.pdf (accessed on 1 March 2020).
3. Home Care for Patients with COVID-19 Presenting with Mild Symptoms and Management of Their Contacts. Available online: https://www.who.int/publications-detail/home-care-for-patients-with-suspected-novel-coronavirus-(ncov)-infection-presenting-with-mild-symptoms-and-management-of-contacts (accessed on 1 March 2020).
4. Irwin, R.R.J. *Intensive Care Medicine*; Lippincott Williams & Wilkins: London, UK, 2008; p. 6.
5. Bolton, R.; Bleetman, A. Non-invasive ventilation and continuous positive pressure ventilation in emergency departments: Where are we now? *Emerg. Med. J.* **2008**, *25*, 190–194. [CrossRef] [PubMed]
6. COVID-19 Italia. Available online: http://opendatadpc.maps.arcgis.com/apps/opsdashboard/index.html#/dae18c330e8e4093bb090ab0aa2b4892 (accessed on 1 March 2020).
7. EASY COVID 19. Available online: https://www.isinnova.it/easy-covid19/ (accessed on 1 March 2020).
8. Autorizzazione all'uso Compassionevole di Dispositivi Medici Privi di Marcatura CE per la Destinazione d'uso Richiesta. Available online: http://www.salute.gov.it/portale/ministro/p4_8_0.jsp?lingua=italiano&label=servizionline&idMat=DM&idAmb=UC&idSrv=A1&flag=P (accessed on 28 March 2020).
9. COVID-19 Call to Action–Connecting People in Need with Those who can Help Using Advanced Digital Manufacturing Solutions. Available online: https://www.3dsystems.com/covid-19-response#signUp (accessed on 1 April 2020).
10. Furlow, B. Medical 3-D Printing. *Radiol. Technol.* **2017**, *88*, 519CT–537CT. [PubMed]
11. Crivello, J.V.; Reichmanis, E. Photopolymer Materials and Processes for Advanced Technologies. *Chem. Mater.* **2014**, *26*, 533–548. [CrossRef]
12. Ligon, S.C.; Liska, R.; Stampfl, J.; Gurr, M.; Mülhaupt, R. Polymers for 3D Printing and Customized Additive Manufacturing. *Chem. Rev.* **2017**, *117*, 10212–10290. [CrossRef] [PubMed]
13. Örtorp, A.; Jemt, T. CNC-milled titanium frameworks supported by implants in the edentulous jaw: A 10-year comparative clinical study. *Clin. Implant Dent. Relat. Res.* **2012**, *14*, 88–99. [CrossRef] [PubMed]
14. Montanini, R.; Scafidi, M.; Staiti, G.; Marcianò, A.; D'Acquisto, L.; Oteri, G. Misfit evaluation of implant supported metal frameworks manufactured with different techniques: Photoelastic and strain gauge measurements. *Proc. Inst. Mech. Eng. Part H J. Eng. Med.* **2016**, *230*, 1106–1116. [CrossRef]
15. Peditto, M.; Nucera, R.; Rubino, E.; Marcianò, A.; Bitto, M.; Catania, A.; Oteri, G. Improving Oral Surgery: A Workflow Proposal to Create Custom 3D Templates for Surgical Procedures. *Open Dent. J.* **2020**, *14*, 35–44. [CrossRef]
16. Fiorillo, L.; D'Amico, C.; Turkina, A.Y.; Nicita, F.; Amoroso, G.; Risitano, G. Endo and Exoskeleton: New Technologies on Composite Materials. *Prosthesis* **2020**, *2*, 1–9. [CrossRef]
17. Cicciù, M. *Prosthesis*: New Technological Opportunities and Innovative Biomedical Devices. *Prosthesis* **2019**, *1*, 1–2. [CrossRef]

© 2020 by the authors. Licensee MDPI, Basel, Switzerland. This article is an open access article distributed under the terms and conditions of the Creative Commons Attribution (CC BY) license (http://creativecommons.org/licenses/by/4.0/).

MDPI
St. Alban-Anlage 66
4052 Basel
Switzerland
Tel. +41 61 683 77 34
Fax +41 61 302 89 18
www.mdpi.com

Prosthesis Editorial Office
E-mail: prosthesis@mdpi.com
www.mdpi.com/journal/prosthesis

www.ingramcontent.com/pod-product-compliance
Lightning Source LLC
LaVergne TN
LVHW070542100526
838202LV00012B/357